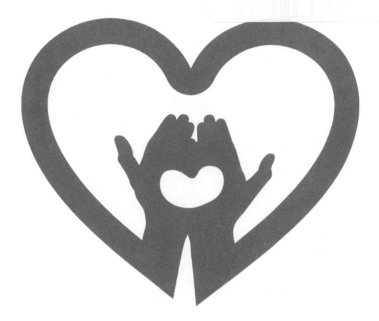

MY NEW KIDNEY & ME

A PKD Patient's Transplant Story

GREG BALDAUF

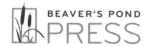
Beaver's Pond
PRESS

Edited by Wendy Weckwerth.

ISBN 13: 978-1-64343-982-2
Library of Congress Catalog Number: 2019906165
Printed in the United States of America
First Printing: 2020
24 23 22 21 20   5 4 3 2 1

Cover and interior design by Dan Pitts.

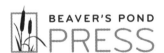

Beaver's Pond Press, Inc.
939 Seventh Street West
Saint Paul, MN 55102
(952) 829-8818
www.BeaversPondPress.com

To order, visit www.ItascaBooks.com or call (800) 901-3480.
Reseller discounts available.

Contact Greg Baldauf at www.GregsNewKidney.com for speaking engagements, book club discussions, and interviews.

For Audrey, Sarah, Emily, and Luke.

For Bret and all organ donors who have restored life—
and to all those who have tried.

For all who suffer from polycystic kidney disease (PKD)
and the family members and friends who support them.

Then, like a radiant star
The Angel of Death
The Angel of Life became
And transformed my dream
From a drama of fear
To a joyful comedy

—Miguel Ángel Ruiz, "Return to Life"

TABLE OF CONTENTS

PROLOGUE

My kidney transplant story is a privileged one, filled with wonder and concluding in a happy ending. Yes, my medical journey had an *extremely* positive outcome—but it was a long, challenging road.

What happened to me and my family throughout a twenty-two-month process—discovering I was in renal failure, needing a kidney transplant, searching for a donor, having the surgery, and recovering—made for a remarkable experience and now, I hope, for a useful and interesting book. This is the saga of struggling against the betrayal of my body, facing my own vulnerability, and learning what it means to confront and overcome life-threatening adversity.

As my story begins, I was living a reasonably ordinary life. I was a husband, a father of three, and a fifty-nine-year-old professor of counseling and psychology at a community college. Thankfully the earlier excitement of my thirties and forties was seemingly long past. Thinking about the end of my teaching career and retirement was the only concern on my radar. Overall, I was content and reasonably happy.

Born in Chicago, I grew up as one of four kids in a northern Chicago suburb called Morton Grove. My wife, Audrey, was raised at the other end of the greater Chicago area, in Plainfield. We met in 1969 at Southern Illinois University when we were both freshmen. From there it was on to Evanston, Illinois, where Audrey went to nursing school and I completed my undergraduate degree at Northwestern University. With a few hiccups and interruptions in between, we raised our family in Evanston over the next thirty-plus years.

So there we were. I was teaching at Oakton Community College, and Audrey was a certified registered nurse anesthetist (CRNA) at the community hospital in Evanston. Our kids, Sarah, Luke, and Emily, then ranging in age from twenty-two to thirty-five, were each finding their paths in the greater world. We were living a pretty good life: fulfilling jobs, an active lifestyle, friends, travel, and the joy of knowing our children as grown-ups.

I was teaching classes in psychology and human services, coordinating the human services and substance-abuse programs, and acting as a counselor at the college. Since my early forties, I'd been studying the ways of indigenous peoples from the Andes of South America. This led to some deeply inspiring trips to Peru, where I was privileged to learn from the *paqos* (shamans) and medicine people—knowledge I drew on at many stages of my illness and recovery.

With retirement a couple of years on the horizon, Audrey and I had started planning a move to Venice, Florida, where several of our couple friends had happily relocated. Our future looked bright. There was just one problem: polycystic kidney disease (PKD), a lifelong health challenge, caught up with me.

No one avoids struggle and pain. I'm no exception. As our bodies wear out, we gradually learn that life consists of tragedies, small and large. In my particular case, it felt as if my body betrayed me. But, ironically, a devastating turn of events led to incredibly good fortune, grace, and unexpected discoveries. The transplant experience enhanced my awareness of who I am as a person and delivered profound gifts along the road from medical trauma to renewed health.

I'm thankful I experienced an excellent outcome in the risky world of organ transplants. Many others have also fared well after getting a new kidney, but in that context "faring well" is difficult to define. It ranges from just being alive to getting off dialysis—or even reaching a level of recovery that allows normal, age-appropriate functioning. Every person with PKD or another kidney-damaging illness has a different story to tell about transplantation and the struggles and complexities that go with it. Those who waited years for a transplant, were ravaged by diabetes, or were on dialysis for years rarely have the positive outcome I'm enjoying.

Patients who need a transplant often wait four to five years before an organ becomes available. The time a person waits to get a kidney varies from state to state and hospital to hospital, and it can be influenced by the patient living in a rural or urban area. Meanwhile, the length of time a person is on dialysis can dramatically affect his or her overall health. According to staff members at the Transplant Clinic at the University of Chicago (UChicago) Medicine, for every month a person is on dialysis, life expectancy can potentially drop by about a year.

Even after transplant surgery, the patient is still at risk; about 5 percent of transplant patients reject the kidneys they receive for various medical reasons. About 20 percent of transplant patients go through at least one immune-system episode in which the threat of rejection comes seriously into play. In organ transplantation, numerous factors can go wrong—or terribly wrong—jeopardizing the patient's health and recovery.

An illustration of such potential complications comes from Audrey's career in operating rooms. Two patients with PKD arrived the same week in the operating room where she was assigned. Both were women in their thirties who'd had kidney transplants, but now needed surgery for transplant-related issues. One was rejecting the kidney, and the other was having her old polycystic kidneys removed because of the pain they were causing. These types of issues aren't infrequent. I'm acutely aware now that organ transplants are not *natural*. Transplants are medical and scientific miracles that prolong life for those fortunate to receive them. But the gift of transplantation comes with strings attached, such as a lifetime of taking immunosuppressing drugs and shouldering the risks that come with those medications.

My story, despite its idiosyncratic twists and turns, intersects with all transplant patients. The process forges a common bond among us. Specific medical complications or nuances aside, all organ-transplant patients—kidney, pancreas, heart, lung, etc.—share characteristic experiences. We walk similar paths through the minefield leading to the actual organ transplant: a severe medical issue that requires a drastic intervention; the wait or search, or both, for a donor (living or deceased); the recovery process from transplant surgery; and then the struggle of coping and living with antirejection medications for the remainder of our lives.

What's unique to PKD patients is that our illness is the largest and most underrecognized genetic disease in the United States. In a 2012 letter to me, Suzanne F. Ruff, author of *The Reluctant Donor*, wrote:

> Polycystic kidney disease (PKD) is the most common, life-threatening genetic disease. More than 600,000 Americans and 12.5 million people worldwide have the disease. It is more common than Down syndrome, cystic fibrosis, muscular dystrophy, sickle cell anemia, hemophilia, and Huntington's disease—*combined*.

As a result of this ignorance about the disease itself, PKD is often shrouded in mystery and, sadly, secrecy in families. It certainly was in my family of origin.

My younger daughter, Emily, who got involved as a volunteer fundraiser with the Northeast Ohio Chapter of the PKD Foundation, recounted a fellow volunteer confessing she'd known nothing about the disease until her father announced at their Sunday family dinner that he was having a kidney transplant the following week because he was in PKD-related renal failure. I've learned this isn't an entirely infrequent way to find out about PKD. Although information about PKD is more readily available now than when I or my family members received transplants, the disease still isn't well known or understood by the general public, and people stricken with PKD and their families often don't know what to do. They're forced to start from square one—ignorance and confusion—when the disease suddenly becomes critical to an individual and his or her family.

As you might expect, PKD research hasn't benefited from the level of financial support given to better-known diseases, such as cancer and heart disease. Charitable donations tend to go to mainstream charities with name recognition and excellent marketing strategies. (According to Charity Navigator, in 2016–17, the PKD Foundation raised $5,419,922 for research and education. In that same period, the American Cancer Society raised $363,786,884, and the American Heart Association raised $269,793,029.) The task for those suffering from PKD isn't only to raise more funds for medical research, but also to raise awareness so people and families coping with PKD can be better served and their disease better treated—and to increase the number of living donors.

PKD has a complicated history in my family. Even though my father, George, and his siblings—a sister and two brothers—had the disease, this information was cloaked in mystery and secrets. From my vantage point as an adolescent, PKD was hidden and rarely discussed. The afflicted family members rarely spoke of it, perhaps because any illness or disease was perceived as weakness. Any discussion of PKD was rare and in hushed tones. Only occasional overheard phone conversations or interactions at family gatherings gave me any inkling that PKD was ravaging my family.

For example, for years I assumed Uncle Carl, the first person in the extended Baldauf family to admit he had the disease, had received a kidney transplant. Only during my own fight with PKD did I learn from my cousin Sharon Gitzen (a wonderful resource and comfort to me throughout my experience) that her dad didn't actually receive a transplant. Furthermore, my dad's youngest brother, Bill, the sibling he was closest to, didn't even know my dad had PKD.

Family cultures look strange when examined closely and objectively. PKD—a little-known, life-threatening illness with no known cure—makes them appear even stranger. Fortunately, the family culture changed significantly in my generation—we've come out of hiding. Hopefully, my children's generation will continue that trend. With ongoing efforts to bring the disease out of quiet corners and into more open discussion, future PKD patients and their families will share a common knowledge about the disease. And with new research, PKD patients will enjoy full lives with a reduced risk of experiencing transplantation.

The core of this book is a step-by-step description of the ordeal I faced as I confronted PKD and had a kidney transplant. In that sense, it's an individual's story. But it reflects a larger story experienced by many others who have faced a life-threatening disease and had a transplant. The PKD struggle for individuals and their families requires courage, tenacity, and optimism when the disease becomes acute. I hope my story will help people in the same situation and assist their family members to cope, survive, and even thrive.

In the case of PKD, the family suffers and struggles as much or more than the kidney recipient, since most support goes to the patient. Motivated by the secrecy around PKD in my extended family, I'm working hard to be candid about my experience—no secrets, no silence, no hiding. Living as a post-transplant PKD patient, I'm committed to telling my truth about what I experienced—with the hope of helping to end the mystery of PKD and the fear surrounding it.

This book also bears witness to how one person chose to confront adversity when his life exploded. Most of us will experience a time when "the wolves are at the door." Sometimes the danger enters dramatically, sometimes insidiously. This isn't a story limited to navigating a physical or medical breakdown. In the largest sense, it's about how one man, backed by a superstar team of family and supporters, confronted a crisis that threatened disability or even death.

One of the most crucial things I learned was how my attitudes influenced my journey. Choosing to open my mind and heart permitted me to recognize the gifts afforded me during my struggle and experience tremendous gratitude as a result. I wasn't just fighting for my health and well-being. I was living life fully, passionately, and deeply in ways I hadn't before. Confronting a life-threatening disease and receiving an organ transplant inevitably bring transformation— and being given one's life back offers a tremendous opening for self-examination and enhanced awareness. But as with all opportunities for transformation, the person has to answer the call, respond, and be open to the vast potential that exists in facing crisis and conflict. My transplant experience was a gift that enhanced and enriched my life. Along the way, I've also come to believe that the opportunity for transformation exists for the donor as well.

I encourage you—the reader, the transplant patient, or the transplant patient's family member—to read this book with an open mind, a beginner's mind. Using a "beginner's mind" means looking at a situation as completely new, leaving behind previous biases or assumed knowledge that could interfere with a present assessment. A beginner's mind not only enhances what can be gained but allows a transplant patient (or someone with PKD or someone who knows someone with PKD) to approach and deal with the situation as creatively and effectively as possible. Using a beginner's mind from the start enriches your experience and helps you to cope and grow—emotionally, psychologically, and spiritually—from your process and your recovery. It also can increase your chance of a positive, successful outcome.

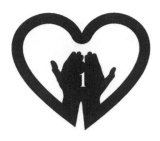

BOOM GOES THE DYNAMITE: A HARSH DOSE OF REALITY

The truth is cruel, but it can be loved,
and it makes free those who have loved it.

—GEORGE SANTAYANA

With the directness of a falling ax, my life—which was fairly typical for a middle-class, white male in his late fifties—turned upside down. The familiar and secure recoiled. My greatest fear—kidney failure—was suddenly true. The cosmic screw turned, and in the time it took to casually retrieve a voice-mail message from my nephrologist's nurse, Jaung, my worst nightmare became my new reality. I was in renal failure. December 17, 2010, will live in infamy.

I was catapulted into the world of renal failure and all its gloominess. Ugh. I needed a kidney transplant because of polycystic kidney disease (PKD), the growth of cysts on the kidneys that gradually impedes their functioning. PKD is a genetic medical condition I'd lived with all my life, but in many ways I knew very little about it. I used avoidance and denial to protect myself from acknowledging the fragile nature of my health. On the rare occasions when I mentally or emotionally acknowledged I had PKD and its attendant health risks, I did so gingerly . . . and briefly. I could only allow myself glimpses of how terrifying kidney failure and transplant surgery could be. My well-worn strategy came to a sudden halt when I listened to the phone message.

Since being introduced to PKD in my adolescence by family members suffering from it, I cultivated and nurtured the fantasy that a kidney transplant would *not* become my reality. My magical thinking was strong. I'd staunchly resisted my nephrologist's words five years earlier when he'd said, "It's not *if*, it's *when* you'll need a transplant." *But what if . . . ?* I thought and perhaps even said that day in his office. Dr. Kevin Nash shrugged, not wanting to crush my spirit entirely. But he knew. His words were prophetic. My wife, Audrey, and I left his office that day with a tad bit of hope, but also with a harsh new reality creeping into our lives.

Vividly recalling that visit, I returned Nurse Jaung's call. She was alarmed and concerned as she reported the results of my blood work: "Your creatinine is 6.0." I was floored. Creatinine levels in the blood are the primary indicator of healthy or problematic kidney function. A high creatinine level means the kidneys aren't successfully performing their job of filtering toxins out of the bloodstream. This high level of 6.0 was a dramatic increase from the 3.5 on my last lab test fifteen months earlier. That was a long time for a patient with PKD to go without a blood test and an indication of my avoidance. I was very committed to the fantasy of that 3.5 number never changing. A creatinine of 6.0 far exceeded the dreaded 4.0—the *number of no return* when a nephrologist recommends you get on a donor list and contact a kidney transplant center. A creatinine test result of 4.0 is an absolute marker in the world of kidney transplantation. And I had vaulted well past that to 6.0.

Jaung proceeded to ask me a series of questions. There was urgency in her voice. "Are you in pain?"

"No."

"Are you light-headed?"

"No."

"Has there been blood in your urine?"

"Never."

On she went, determined to do her job. Other than the high blood pressure I treated successfully for thirty-five years, I had no symptoms or issues with my PKD. I was slightly relieved to keep answering her queries in the negative. If I said *no* often enough, perhaps I could win her over. Maybe she would revoke the bad news and accept that this lab test was obviously a fluke. My denial was strong enough to make me think I could even overcome medical data by force of will.

I finally interrupted. "I just got in from working out at the gym for an hour and a half. I feel a little tired at the moment but overall very good. Even great."

She paused but remained firmly committed to her data-based convictions. She recommended I make an appointment and have my blood drawn again.

I agreed. Surely the second test would prove the first an anomaly. I scheduled a doctor's appointment for January, after the holidays. Was there a glimmer of hope? Maybe, but deep down the forged-steel foundation of my denial was irrevocably cracked. I felt a slight shift in my reality, hardly perceptible, but nonetheless one that couldn't be altered or reversed. My disavowal of degenerative PKD was fractured. Soon it would be shattered entirely.

Stunned by the phone conversation with the nurse, I anxiously paced around the den. I was in shock. Not knowing what to do, my mind raced and my heart pounded. I was on the edge of panic. It was like I was in a dream state or having an out-of-body experience. I was watching myself and my thoughts like I was in a movie. *What the hell just happened? If this is true, I'm screwed.*

Dazed, confused, and rattled, I did the only thing I knew to do. I picked up the phone and called Audrey. Calling her at work was significant because, as a nurse anesthetist working in an operating room, she's responsible for keeping a patient alive and breathing during surgery. Phoning necessitated some deliberation about whether my news was truly important. With a wry smile (one's true character always presents itself), I decided it just might be.

Audrey had been sharing my PKD story and the possibility of a kidney transplant for more than forty years. I relied on her as wife, partner, lover, and friend to support me living with PKD. She shared my resolute belief that I could make it to old age without a transplant. Audrey kept me grounded, contributing information and insights and helping me stay in the vicinity of reality regarding my kidneys.

With a quiver in my voice, I told her what had transpired.

"How do you feel?" she asked. "Maybe it's a bad lab."

We were partners in our shared conviction. She didn't want to completely surrender our shared fantasy either. She was empathetic, but I recognized her worry. She knew what crossing the threshold of a 4.0 creatinine level meant. When I hung up the phone and sat down, I was muttering and punctuating my ramblings with numerous expletives. I could barely wait until she got home.

I was terrified. Behind my outburst of raw emotions that filled my time waiting, I realized I was thinking about my older brother, Tom—who had died at age fifty, about fifteen years earlier, from complications associated with PKD and a transplant. Memories of him and his suffering flooded in. Tom and I were the "unfortunate ones" in our immediate family. We had PKD. It is a fifty-fifty genetic flip of the coin that determines who gets PKD (assuming one parent has the gene). Of my parents' four children—Jerry, Tom, me, and Roseann— Tom and I lost the coin flip.

Tom had a kidney transplant in 1982 when he was thirty-five. His transplant lasted fifteen years, which in that era was quite remarkable. Tom suffered through the dark ages of organ transplants. Kidney transplants were just out of their toddlerhood if not infancy in 1982, although the first kidney transplant in the world was done in Chicago at Little Company of Mary Hospital in 1950 on Ruth Tucker, a PKD patient. She survived for four months. (According to the National Kidney Center, the first *successful* transplant was performed on identical twins in Boston in 1954.) The thirty-five or so different medications Tom required was extreme by today's medical standards. It was a mind-boggling amount of drugs, which is an apropos description since some of them were "mind benders." His thinking and behavior were sometimes erratic. Physically, his body appeared distorted and misshapen, mostly from the steroids. As his "new" kidney wore out, his bones became necrotic, resulting in two hip replacements. As he lay in a hospital bed dying, the bones in both of his ankles and feet were crumbling. When he died, the doctors said his "heart exploded." Although not sophisticated medically, those words graphically communicated an appalling death.

My family's history of PKD covers the entire spectrum of the disease process. Many were spared the PKD gene—two of my children, two of my siblings, and some first cousins. While my father and two of his siblings who had PKD died of causes that can't be attributed to the disease, Uncle Carl essentially died from renal failure due to PKD. Some of us have had transplants—my aunt Marge Bencivenga, my cousins Sharon Gitzen and Jack Baldauf (after mine in 2017), and Tom and me. Of that group, only Jack and I remain. Through the generations, the saga is ongoing. My son, Luke, has the disease as does my nephew Jon Baldauf. How different the lives of Carl and Tom were to Bill, my uncle with PKD who thrived until he passed away at age ninety of heart failure. In one way or another, PKD has taken a toll on everyone in our family, and evidently it will continue to do so.

Waiting for Audrey to get home, I was overwhelmed by my emotions, but fear and trepidation dominated. Thinking about Tom caused more anxiety. Even though I knew transplant procedures had advanced significantly (largely connected to more effective medications), and that I was substantially healthier than my brother, in those first few hours, medical advancements didn't matter. Logic and rational thinking couldn't soothe me.

I was overwhelmed with ominous questions: *What the hell is going to happen to me? Will I be sick and unable to keep living the life I've known? Will I be on dialysis? Am I going to die?* My ego was disintegrating as my brother's distorted face stared at me. What terrified me the most was being chronically sick or physically diminished. Dialysis was also a horrifying prospect; the idea of a having port in my body for a machine to clean my blood three times a week brought me to my knees. I had never felt more vulnerable. Little did I know that vulnerability would become my almost constant companion over the next twenty-two months.

I know "shit happens" to everyone. Even though I was trying to contextualize that day's bad news as a part of the larger human experience, I felt defeated. I had escaped the evils of PKD for a long time, but renal failure would now advance rapidly. PKD was about to dictate all aspects of my life. The phone call was just the first hit. But somehow I was still standing, if a bit wobbly.

Thirty years earlier, when I first visited my brother's nephrologist as a precautionary measure, he told me I had a degenerative disease. At thirty, *degenerative* didn't really resonate. *Sure I do*, I thought. *How interesting.* Now the disease was suddenly very real and along with *degenerative*, a litany of scary terms was running through my mind: *less than*, *decayed*, *sick*, and, heaven forbid, *dying*. In clinical terms, my condition was called "end-stage renal disease." The reality of it was chilling.

As I waited, the rapid-fire questions renewed: *How bad off am I? Who will donate a kidney? Will someone save me?* The only certainty was that my life had changed. My usual optimism turned to fear. Not knowing what was going to happen created a state of anxiety that would stay present for the next two years.

In retrospect, I recognize that I was swimming (or drowning) in the waters of loss. I was exhibiting three of the five stages of loss that Elisabeth Kübler-Ross articulated some fifty years ago in her

1969 book *On Death and Dying:* denial, anger, and bargaining. In those first hours after receiving the news, my response to the loss of my health was straight out of a fantasy. I was fighting to preserve the life I'd known so far and the life I envisioned for the next thirty years. Looking back, the upside of my mental gymnastics was that I believed I had a life worth living.

POLYCYSTIC KIDNEY DISEASE (PKD)

Normal kidneys filter out excess toxins, waste substances, and fluid from the blood. In people with PKD, the kidneys become enlarged with multiple cysts that interfere with normal function. This interference can lead to renal failure and the need for dialysis or kidney transplantation.

According to the *Medifocus Guidebook on: Polycystic Kidney Disease* (2018), PKD is the most common life-threatening genetic disorder caused by a single gene, and it affects between one in four hundred to one thousand people worldwide. It's characterized by fluid-filled cysts that form in the nephrons (filters) of both kidneys and eventually lead to kidney failure in the majority of patients. PKD is the fourth most common cause of kidney failure.

The blister-like cysts caused by PKD range from the size of a pinhead to as large as a grapefruit. PKD patients may have hundreds or thousands of cysts, which lead to the kidney expanding up to the size of a football and weighing up to thirty-eight pounds.

Hypertension (high blood pressure) is the most common and often the first symptom of PKD. Untreated high blood pressure can cause further kidney damage, while treatment can help slow and might even prevent kidney failure. According to the National Kidney Foundation, other symptoms include back or side pain, an increase in the size of the abdomen, blood in the urine, and frequent bladder or kidney infections.

PKD affects between six hundred thousand and seven hundred thousand people in the United States and approximately 12.5 million people worldwide. Seven to 10 percent of the people on dialysis are believed to be suffering from this disease. The National Kidney Foundation states that PKD is found in all races (and at a slightly higher rate among African Americans) and occurs equally in men and women. It causes about 5 percent of all kidney failure. Other important facts about PKD include:

- Five thousand to six thousand new cases of PKD are diagnosed each year in the United States.

- Forty percent of the cases diagnosed yearly in the United States are people forty-five years old or younger.

- Between 5 and 10 percent of patients diagnosed have no known familial history of PKD.

- About 50 percent of patients diagnosed with autosomal dominant PKD (ADPKD) progress to end-stage renal disease by the age of sixty.

Source: *Medifocus Guidebook on: Polycystic Kidney Disease*, 2018.

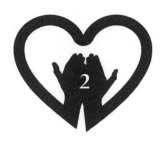

SHARING THE NEWS

The sharing of bad news makes us all children.

—ANONYMOUS

After struggling alone for a few hours, it was good to hear Audrey come through the door. We gripped each other in a bear hug, trying to squeeze the abrasive horror out of the day's incomprehensible news. It worked for a moment, long enough to ground us for what was starting—a long, demanding fight.

The concerned look on her face and the heaviness of her energy were palpable. For my benefit, she stepped up big time. She transcended her own needs and became pure love, concern, and support. Somehow, she flipped the switch in her brain that allowed her to allay her own fears and concentrate on helping me cope and survive. Our more than forty years together have demonstrated that by nature I'm more optimistic, while she's more pessimistic. In that moment, she valiantly suppressed her natural tendencies for doubt and worry. Bolstered by her efforts, some of my natural optimism was briefly restored. Feeling protected and safe, the reprieve I sought was granted. A strong, seemingly impermeable solidarity formed between us in those first few hours. Our existing bond was reinvigorated. Its strength served us well in the coming months.

Audrey's career as a certified registered nurse anesthetist (CRNA), or an advanced practice nurse, had been a blessing to our family and friends over the years. She was a wealth of knowledge and information about hospitals and medical procedures. It was commonplace for her to guide people through the mysteries of the medical world, translate the confusion, help decrease the fear, and make the passage easier. Friends often asked Audrey to recommend a doctor or surgeon. At first, these requests flattered her ego, but over time, she also felt a heavy burden of responsibility. What if her recommendation didn't pan out well? She began sidestepping the inquiries and limiting her involvement to more general advice.

Knowledge can truly be a blessing and a curse. Knowing what really happens in hospitals and how they succeed or fail carries a liability for the knower. I didn't realize until much later what Audrey went through, knowing as she did the risks involved in the surgery and recovery from a kidney transplant. Even now I doubt I grasp everything she knew about the gravity of my condition. My awareness of the risks and severity were usually delivered on a need-to-know basis. Audrey was a buffer, protecting me from being completely overwhelmed— but serving as a shield has a cost.

I frequently thought about the saying my daughter Sarah's husband, Chris Fickes, would offer up when a heated discussion would arise about politics, sports, or culture during a family gathering: "All things will be revealed." How true these words would turn out to be for me during the transplant journey. Medical facts and information, survival tips, insights and, most of all, an awareness of life and healing were revealed to me sporadically, frequently, and sometimes continuously.

Submerging ourselves in the fear, Audrey and I talked, processed, questioned, and talked more. We started to find solace in an emergent belief that we could deal with the challenges that lay ahead. We decided to put our trust in the power of our shared belief system and in each other. Fear, apathy, and anxiety wouldn't be allowed to overwhelm or paralyze us—and certainly not to overtake or defeat us—even if the situation worsened. We would fight and struggle. That day, we committed to a workmanlike approach to this horrible adversity that confronted us and threatened to ruin our lives.

Love and trust allow our strengths to take over rather than our weaknesses. This is not to say weakness and fear were vanquished entirely. But we agreed aloud—and in unspoken telepathic, spiritual, and energetic ways—to take on the challenges and rise to the occasion. Our pact was built on love, mutual trust, and strength, and it created a spontaneous courage that sprung from our truer and better natures. It was our shared triumph of the human spirit. At some deeper level, flowing under our wish-fueled denial, we'd always known a kidney transplant was in our future. The future had just arrived earlier than we'd planned.

Audrey is my most significant gift and blessing. She stemmed the tide of defeat early in my ordeal. As we stumbled through the initial shock and confusion, she set a tone of strength, promise, and hope. Knowing you aren't alone is a powerful elixir. We could have turned in the opposite direction—to despair. Instead, fortified by her strength and our bond in those first few hours and days, we moved forward.

Sounds good, right? Our soulful alliance was profound and a wonderful anchor for what was to come. But a starker reality was merely days away. Our new attitude was going to be tested when our children came home for the holidays. I dreaded telling them, but Audrey dreaded it even more. In recent years, our children had asked more questions about my PKD, especially since I started seeing a nephrologist regularly five years earlier to help track the progress of my disease. After a doctor visit, I'd call or email them with my current creatinine number, blood pressure, and any change in medication. The news had always been generally good, so typically there was little to talk about. Even so, my reports were met with skepticism.

"Are you sure everything is all right?" one of them would ask.

I would counter, "Trust me. I'll let you know when something gets serious."

These exchanges eventually escalated to them expecting a call the day of my visit or labs. All in all, a relative calm had prevailed, but the uneasy peace was about to rudely change. The tariff had come due on my comment that I would tell them when something was serious.

The kids were due home for Christmas in less than a week. How was I going to tell them about my failing kidneys? Their raw emotions were my biggest concern. It was one thing to confront my own fears or Audrey's; it was another to deal with the fears of my daughters and son. *How ironic*, I thought. *Parents protect their children, even their adult children, from harm and injury the best they can, right?* We were about to break this implied sacred oath of parenting and child-rearing to deliver some threatening news.

Telling the kids became our focus—immediate and pressure packed. "What the hell?" we said after an initial gnashing of teeth. "We might as well start the holiday season with something difficult." Gallows humor rarely let us down.

As best we could, we wanted to be honest and forthright with Sarah, Emily, and Luke. Telling the truth was important, especially regarding my PKD. Obviously, my health and well-being were front and center at the moment. But because PKD is a genetic disease, my children's health and lives were also in play. Did they have PKD? Would their children have the disease?

All of the kids were still at risk to have PKD even though, at the time, they were symptom-free. Sarah and Emily had been tested almost twenty years earlier. The jury was still out on Luke's condition at the time of my crisis (later we discovered he has PKD). Our daughters were considering having children. These circumstances increased the tension around our disclosure, making sharing the news even more daunting. The intimacy required and the grittiness of this kind of human exchange made our pending encounter tense and taut. We were about to enter one of the deepest, most fundamental, and terrifying aspects of the human condition: the threat of disease, dying, and death. My renal failure forced us to engage these demons. It felt far too real for ordinary people like us to confront. What was about to happen was a scene you might see in a movie. Only it wouldn't be on celluloid this time. The situation was playing out in our lives . . . and it was painfully real.

We always eagerly anticipate the kids return home during the holiday season. (The truth be told, we feel a similar delight when they return to their own lives a week or so later. A sentiment I believe they share.) We enjoy our Christmas traditions—opening presents Christmas morning, Christmas brunch, and attending the best play available in Chicago a few days later, followed by an extravagant dinner at Smith & Wollensky, a steakhouse in downtown Chicago. From there we'd look down State Street, across the State Street Bridge, to a startling view of the Chicago Theatre ablaze in red and white lights. What an incredible way to celebrate family and the holidays.

Audrey and I swore to protect Christmas morning. But we knew the truth of the matter must prevail. Pretending for too long wouldn't work. Deception, even with the best of intentions, was unacceptable. Despite the strong, ever-present pull of avoidance, honesty and love would serve us in our current situation and in the long run. We believed that once we collectively overcame the shock, the truth and our shared love would help form an unbreakable bond among us.

But the actual reveal to Sarah, Emily, and Luke, along with Sarah's husband, Chris, and Terry Parmelee, Emily's fiancé, was handled poorly. It lacked grace and courage. Honestly, I failed miserably. I deflected the pain of the situation and avoided as much as I could. The delivery of the news really didn't reflect the energy and concern Audrey and I put into our preparation. Fear and anxiety won, and we crashed and burned.

We waited until the day after Christmas. Overall, the morning started quite routinely. We knew that after the natural fatigue of the homecoming and holiday, it was not a bad idea for everyone to separate for a while and relax. The day after Christmas was when we all intuitively knew to go to our separate corners to recharge before our upcoming adventure in the city.

Everyone slowly assembled in the den that morning, snacking and drinking coffee. Our collective weariness was apparent. The kids were sprawled all about on the couches, chairs, and floor. This was the moment I chose to blurt, "I'm going to need a kidney transplant. My blood tests last week said my creatinine was 6.0." The bomb dropped and then exploded. As the shock of my words hit each of them, there was confusion in their eyes. It was followed by silence. A deafening quiet hung in the room. Then tears . . . lots of them. Puzzled looks painted their faces. Worried comments filled the room. Then gloom replaced the earlier carefree tone of the morning.

I don't remember all the commotion and questions that followed. Maybe I've blocked the memories. Perhaps Sarah, the oldest, said, "Wait. What does this mean?" I do remember—as if it were happening right now—the heaviness and sadness that filled the room. I felt like a deer in headlights. It was too much to bear. Sarah and Emily cried. Luke looked shocked and remained silent (a posture he frequently adopted). Chris and Terry watched their partners, not knowing what to say or do. We briefly tried to talk—perhaps stammered and muttered is a better characterization. Then I said, "We're going to go work out. We'll be back in an hour or so. We can talk some more later."

The interaction still seems like a hit-and-run accident. Share the bad news and get the hell out. "What?!" they muttered. But what could they do? I needed to escape the intensity of the situation. I hoped talking with each other without me there might be a good thing.

There's no good way to share terrible news with the people you love the most. I wish I'd done it better. But we did recover. The necessary conversations were had. Questions were asked and answered to the best of our ability. There were tears and hugs and even a few laughs. Fortunately, any damage I might have done in my awkward telling vanished. We repaired ourselves and each other. Love, care, and support formed a safe container that held us and protected us throughout the entire ordeal and beyond.

I was heartened by how much my children cared. I knew they had my back. Audrey was relieved to know she wasn't carrying the burden alone. Emotionally this was a huge step forward for us. The family catharsis emptied buckets of fear. Absorbing their love and support, however, required that we accept the role reversal of our children caring for us. We were to be takers rather than givers. Traditional parent-child roles were blown to smithereens. This reversal was particularly challenging for me. But given the magnitude of what was happening, I eventually embraced the change and was relieved when I let go. Our encounter was the first dramatic example of how my kidney failure necessitated our being adaptable. Flexibility, regardless of form, was compulsory for survival and success.

The holiday farewells that year were extra sweet as we all turned to a new chapter together.

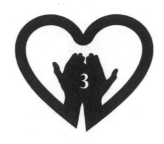

RECONNOITERING

*Once you have begun to distinguish that it's all invented, you
can create a place to dwell where new inventions are the order of
the day. Such a place we call "the universe of possibility."*

—ROSAMUND STONE ZANDER AND BENJAMIN ZANDER,
THE ART OF POSSIBILITY

As was our past practice, Audrey and I went to Florida after the
holidays to enjoy some sun, warmth, and relaxation. A vacation was
a welcome relief from the past weeks' struggles, especially telling
the kids. Because we had done our due diligence telling Sarah, Emily,
and Luke, another upside of this trip was that we could now tell our
friends. Sharing my story broadened our circle of support, and it was
time to take that step. Isolation wouldn't help us.

The love and support offered from our close friends proved
invaluable; it continually lifted our spirits. Alan Rubin, a long-standing
friend, once reminded me that you can't make old friends. This
wisdom proved true as we shared our news, troubles, and worries
over what was happening. Our old friends Jim and Ellen Bush, John
and Pat Tosto, Bernie and Susan Silver, and the new community of
Florida friends contributed significantly to our well-being during that

trip in early 2011. Being in this cradle of care sustained us for what was to come, adding inspiration and strength as I started my journey to find a donor. Time and time again our friends' love and support proved to be essential.

We returned home from Florida peaceful, optimistic, and revived. We stored up as much momentum and hope as possible to use in the months ahead. But a tougher, more threatening, reality awaited us. Vacation was over.

My post-traumatic phone call appointment with Dr. Kevin Nash was on January 12, 2011. He got right to the point. The second blood test confirmed the December results. Wham! Any remnants of hope that the previous lab result was wrong were extinguished. Magical thinking, avoidance, and denial were rendered obsolete. My creatinine was still 6.0. It was game, set, and match. PKD, 6–Greg, 0. This time my test results weren't *probably correct*; they were definitive. It felt life threatening. Hearing Nash confirm what the lab results meant for my medical status felt truly awful. I hit bottom as I realized I was in a fight for my life. Chris's words echoed in my head: "All will be revealed." It was.

Dr. Nash had been recommended to me initially by Audrey, and he was an excellent practitioner. For five years he diligently watched my progress—or, rather, my degeneration. He was my go-to guy for "all things kidney" the last five years: monitoring my condition and medications and conscientiously watching my blood pressure. Now his job expanded; he would keep me alive and as healthy as possible by controlling my levels of vitamin D, phosphate, and potassium. He knew my likely prognosis: renal failure and a transplant. Nash was always forthright while being kind and thoughtful. So far, I'd taken comfort in his approach, but this time his demeanor as he delivered the crushing truth felt somehow nonchalant. He made it eminently clear what end-stage renal disease (ESRD) entailed and what had to happen.

Dr. Nash assigned a short list of big tasks: adjust my medications, pick a transplant center, and get a donor. He wrote prescriptions for new medications to slow the potential damage of renal failure and help protect my other organs and systems. We agreed the primary goal was to keep me off dialysis. Dialysis terrified me. I didn't want to be sick, tired, and physically limited—or dependent on a machine to live. The thought of having a port surgically inserted in my arm to make the dialysis easier made me shiver. I was adamant about this direction of my care. Fortunately, Nash agreed. In fact, he was quite reassuring about it, sharing a story about a previous patient he'd kept off dialysis even though his creatinine was 12.0. The story resonated with me. I didn't realize at the time the full implications of this joint decision or how beneficial avoiding dialysis would be. Nash was good to his word. Avoiding dialysis was a clear example of how crossroads situations, of which there were many, frequently turned in my favor.

We discussed the local and out-of-state transplant centers. He was informative but impartial. Audrey and I leaned toward the University of Chicago hospital, or UChicago Medicine, largely because their residents were rotating through Evanston Hospital and she liked what she saw. Nash worked with patients from most of the area transplant hospitals, so the final decision was ours. We tried to be proactive and assert ourselves at every opportunity. Making decisions empowered us.

In this case, we chose the UChicago Medicine and its Kidney Transplant Clinic, which proved invaluable for my recovery. What a gift the clinic team turned out to be. Having the transplant at UChicago proved to be one of the best choices we made. In retrospect, I can see that a pattern of good fortune was developing.

I had tears in my eyes as we left Nash's office somber, but with some confidence. Our anxiety decreased by having Nash as a partner and developing a plan but increased after his delivery of the unyielding diagnosis itself. A melancholy surfaced as a result, knowing the reality of what I was really dealing with. Things looked ominous, and a heaviness filled us both. Even our attempts to enlist an old friend, gallows humor, hoping it would dispel some of the emotional weight, had limited success.

The whole situation struck us as arbitrary. The enormity of the situation and how tiny we seemed in comparison left us feeling overwhelmed and powerless. We acknowledged how little we knew and questioned our ability to influence the situation. *Would we, could we, get this thing right?* We slowly started to acknowledge our limits and lack of influence. We agreed to work hard, be diligent, and stay committed to the task. We also acknowledged that something beyond our own efforts would be necessary for us to succeed. Random luck, divine intervention, or both would be welcomed and greatly appreciated.

Through the evening and into the next morning, optimism returned. I had a strong sense that when I faced my fears, they were replaced with strength and courage. We affirmed to each other that we could pull this thing off or at least exert a titanic effort to influence a positive outcome. Returning to some semblance of a normal life was attainable. Our attitudes varied and waned in the coming months, sometimes even from minute to minute, hour to hour, and day to day. Throughout, no matter what transpired, we reset to a place of optimism, calm, and stability. How we found the courage and strength remains a mystery, but being able to regain our balance and carry on was crucial to our success.

Our ongoing, heartfelt conversations revealed three central attitudes. The first was that we often felt as if we were on the ocean, where wind and currents influenced our direction more than any effort we could exert. But regardless of precarious conditions or how powerless we felt, we consistently moved forward and stayed the course. Persistence—and the love and support of our family and friends—pushed us forward. I felt I was being carried along on a perilous but somehow protected journey. We made friends with the uncertainty and ambiguity, and learned to embrace a go-with-the-flow approach.

The second attitude was characterized by a sense of strength and optimism. Fashioned by our decision to survive, Audrey and I believed we would prevail. A shared, internal sense of power created a synergy that allowed us to overcome whatever challenges came our way. Our positive attitude was self-reinforcing and contagious. For example, when I'd ask Luke how he was doing with my struggle, he'd reply: "OK. I'm just flowing with how you're responding." When it was reflected back to us by our family and friends, our optimism grew stronger. The struggle to keep going, to navigate the process, became more important than the objectives of finding a donor and having the transplant. The outcomes—getting a kidney, having a transplant, and surviving—weren't the singular focus, which isn't to say we ever lost sight of them. We immersed ourselves in this inherently life-giving process. Engagement was essential, as was acknowledging the process itself as transformative—no matter the outcome. Ironically, my disease was creating an opportunity for learning, growth, and reinvention.

The third prevailing attitude was that there was a spiritual, somehow egoless, quality to this adventure. Something unfamiliar was engaged. I'd never felt quite like this before. I'd experienced moments I called "spiritual," during my time in the Andes working with the Inca paqos and in my relationships, but never when my life or well-being was at risk or held in the balance. Now I was participating in the hero's journey, as Joseph Campbell called it. I was in the middle of an experience that was bigger than me, that was taking me on an unknown journey, the implications of which were broader and more significant than one person's struggles. Struggling to stay alive was expanding my understanding of the essence of being alive.

My experience was influenced by my attitude, choices, and active participation in a demanding and dangerous process. One of my favorite writers, Joan Borysenko, author of *Minding the Body, Mending the Mind,* quotes an old Hindu saying, "God does not remove the flies from a cow's behind unless it moves its tail." Recalling these words reminded me this wasn't the time to be passive, but rather the moment to do everything possible to influence the outcome. One of the reasons I made it to almost sixty before needing a transplant was that I'd been moving my tail. I worked at wellness by trying to stay healthy in mind, body, and spirit.

I embraced the idea that the outcome of my disease wasn't yet determined. It could be influenced by what I did or didn't choose to do. This belief reduced my feeling of having no control at all. There's an extremely thin space between powerlessness and agency when people with sickness and disease walk the tightrope of their predicament. It's a paradox all human beings eventually navigate. We all routinely and regularly engage life most fully between choice and inevitability, but that polarity becomes especially stark when we're confronted with a crisis.

I began to grasp that my situation presented an opportunity. The intensity of my ordeal afforded me an opportunity to live life fully. I started thinking my life-and-death struggle, a fight I didn't choose, was a powerful learning opportunity. Everyday life expanded as I was given a chance to truly live. I was going to fight the fight while maintaining some level of dignity and integrity. When framed this way, the possible outcomes took on different dimensions. The conclusion and the struggle were on equal terms. Of course, I passionately wanted to survive, even flourish. But in the end, survival wasn't the only measure of the worthiness of my efforts.

With all this in mind—bolstered by the love and support of Audrey, my children, and our friends and family—I took the next step. I called UChicago Medicine's Kidney Transplant Clinic to arrange an appointment for an orientation session on February 10, 2011. The donor-transplant mission began in earnest.

Prior to my first visit to the Transplant Clinic, I felt compelled to widen the circle of support. Up to this point, only my family and closest friends knew I was in renal failure. On February 7, 2011, I emailed my two surviving siblings, Jerry Baldauf and Roseann Baldauf-Shales, and my uncle and his wife, Bill and Irene Baldauf:

> I've been meaning to call to tell you this in person,
> but my phone aversion has gotten the best of me.

A blood test in mid-December indicated my kidney function is in trouble. My creatinine went from 3.5 to 6.0 in the last eighteen months. The cutoff is 4.0. My other numbers were also elevated. These numbers were confirmed in a follow-up test last month. No other symptoms yet except some fatigue.

Consequently, starting Thursday, February 10, I'm starting the process to get a kidney transplant at UChicago.

I have an orientation session scheduled on 2/10, and testing and a meeting with the transplant team on 2/16.

Obviously, I'm at the beginning of this process, and I have a lot to learn; but both my doctor and nephrologist recommend that if I can get a donor kidney, I should have the transplant sooner than later. I'm told the average wait on the donor list is two years. And I'd sure like to avoid dialysis by getting one sooner. We'll see . . .

I'll be putting out some kind of request (plea?) for a kidney to everyone I can think of in the near future.

Bill and Irene, I'd like to get Sharon's phone number from you. She's the healthiest transplant patient I know.

This should be an interesting adventure. I'll keep you posted as I find out more.

Love, Greg

When I read that message now, I find it so understated. But it conveys how cautious I was and the power of the conflict I was dealing with those first couple of months. My family members' responses were touching. They moved the discussion right to the question of finding a donor. I emailed them back. Here's my reply to Jerry:

Jer,

Good to hear from you. I wish it was for a better
reason, but be that as it may . . . I'll take it.

I greatly appreciate any and all conversations,
but I certainly understand about your general health
issues. Given what you've said, I doubt you'd be a
strong candidate to cough up a kidney.

I'm not sure "complex" describes the situation.
What's beyond complex? I can tell you it is
extremely weird to be asking others for a body part.
With that said, it is all about a donor at this point.
There's much reason for optimism if I get a good
match and if you consider my overall health and age.
Transplants, especially for kidneys, are light years
ahead of what they were even ten years ago, and the
antirejection drugs are also vastly improved. A far
cry from what Tom went through.

I'd hoped to dodge this bullet and follow Uncle
Bill's path. I guess having gotten to my sixtieth year
isn't too bad—all things considered. My number
just came up.

Anyway, I'm trying to see this as an adventure.
We all get something. I've known this was a
possibility all my life.

I'll be in touch as I find out more.

Love, Greg

When I wrote the initial email to my extended family, I only intended
to inform them of what was happening. I thought it was unlikely that
either of my siblings, due to health reasons, would give me a kidney.
I hadn't anticipated their discussion of giving me a kidney, but clearly
they recognized the priority of finding a donor. As a result of my
emails, Roseann was alerted to possibly being a donor; Jerry became

a constant line of love, support, and humor; and Bill and Irene got me connected with other members of my extended family.

I decided a call to Sharon Gitzen, my first cousin and a transplant recipient, was in order. It was one of the best things I did. She was loving and supportive and a wellspring of information. As a twelve-year transplant veteran, she knew well the details, options, and problems associated with getting a donor, having the surgery, recovering, and living as a transplant patient. Of all the helpful things Sharon said in that first phone call, the one that resonated the most was: "Find a healthy donor; it's really the most important thing." That piece of wisdom ultimately determined my fate eight months later.

At this early stage in the journey, some conscious and unconscious truths had already emerged: I would be loved and supported by my extended family and many others. Finding a donor was paramount; it stood above all else. I had a vast amount to learn about myself. And a significant number of unexpected, hidden gifts awaited me.

ORGAN DONATION

According to the National Kidney Foundation, in 2014, 17,107 kidney transplants took place in the United States. Of these, 11,570 kidney transplants came from deceased donors, and 5,537 came from living donors.

People between the ages of thirty-five and forty-nine were the largest age group to donate among living donors. People between the ages of eighteen and thirty-four constituted the second-largest age group. Donors under fifty years old are considered the healthiest individuals to donate a kidney.

More women than men are living donors: 61.4 percent to 38.6 percent.

Most donors have some familial relationship to the recipient or are a spouse or life partner. Approximately 18 percent are either a nonrelative paired donation or an anonymous donor.

I was very fortunate—among the approximately one in ten recipients—to receive a kidney from a living donor, which according to the UChicago Medicine Kidney Transplant Clinic insures a far better rate of the transplant lasting a longer time.

TYPES OF POLYCYSTIC KIDNEY DISEASES

There are three major forms of PKD: autosomal dominant polycystic kidney disease (ADPKD), autosomal recessive polycystic kidney disease (ARPKD), and acquired cystic kidney disease (ACKD).

ADPKD is the most common hereditary disease; it occurs in approximately one in every four hundred to one thousand people. Each child of an autosomal-dominant affected parent has a 50 percent chance of inheriting the disease, which means it doesn't skip a generation. For example, if a patient with the disease doesn't pass it along to one of his or her children, then the disease disappears from that family, and grandchildren can't inherit the disease. Some patients with ADPKD aren't diagnosed during their lifetime due to a lack of symptoms, which sometimes results in a family member having the disease and not knowing it. In approximately 15 percent of cases, ADPKD occurs in people without a family history of the disease. The appearance of ADPKD is due to the patient having a new genetic mutation that wasn't present in either parent. According to the National Human Genome Research Institute, about half of individuals who have ADPKD develop end-stage kidney disease by the age of sixty.

ARPKD is uncommon and is typically diagnosed in infancy or in utero, with less severe forms being diagnosed later in childhood or adolescence. ARPKD occurs in approximately one in twenty thousand people. The term *recessive* in the disease's name means the mutated gene must be present in both parents. Because each parent has one abnormal and one normal gene, they are considered carriers. There then is a 25 percent chance that each child will inherit an abnormal gene from both parents and have the disease.

ACKD isn't inherited. It develops most commonly in patients who have been on dialysis for five years or longer, and it's found in 20 percent of patients with end-stage renal disease.

Source: *Medifocus Guidebook on: Polycystic Kidney Disease*, 2018.

CROSSING THE THRESHOLD, MAKING THE CONNECTION

We must let go of the life we have planned, so as to accept the one that is waiting for us.

— JOSEPH CAMPBELL

While waiting for the orientation session and acceptance into UChicago's Transplant Center, even without the urgings from my family members, my thinking had turned to finding a donor. Searching for someone to give me an organ was the most nerve-racking, complex, and demanding work of the entire ordeal. That quest was to be the defining task of my life. Threatened, fearful, anxious, terrified, hopeful, and optimistic were the feelings that flooded my awareness and invaded my waking and sleeping hours. The stress was constant. Infrequently, I quieted them by distracting myself. Ultimately, the unending scroll came down to the essential question: *Will I find a kidney donor?*

I was afraid to discover if someone cared enough about me to donate a kidney. My self-worth was in question. I desperately wanted to believe there were people in my life who would donate, but when put to the test, as I was now, I asked myself, *Will it actually happen? Do I deserve to get a donor? Am I good enough?* With karma in mind, I wondered, *Will my past sins and mistakes catch up with me?* My questions were genuine but also irrational. They demonstrated the panic and crazy thinking I was immersed in. I learned over time that being good enough or deserving ultimately had nothing to do with getting a kidney. My need and a donor's ability to give were distinct and separate in many ways, but they hopefully would intersect. I bounced between optimism and fear, with a strong dash of continuous doubt.

Asking for a person's body part was a mind-blowing challenge. Even now, the search long over, the idea of a person giving me a kidney inspires wonder, awe, humility, gratitude, and confusion. My pursuit of a donor became utterly consuming. All else paled in comparison. I was forced to find the wherewithal to not only accept my task but also succeed at it.

Fueled by this sense of urgency, a momentum emerged. I started telling more people what was happening. As I told other friends and extended family members, copious support rolled in. Why people "rise to the occasion" when another is in need is complex, and I'm uncertain of a definitive answer, but the groundswell of support in my life when I needed it the most speaks well of peoples' capacity to love. Comfort and encouragement from others were essential to surviving, and later thriving, as my trial progressed.

Support from family members—particularly from my siblings, Jerry and Roseann—arrived via email. Then shortly after I attended the orientation session, the unexpected happened. My brother-in-law, Al Downs, and my second cousin John Pablocki each offered me a kidney.

Al, the husband of Audrey's sister, Chris, was an unlikely donor because of his age. I was shocked but encouraged by his offer, which left me feeling optimistic about my quest. When it was followed by John's offer, I was flabbergasted. *Holy shit,* I thought, *you've got to be kidding me.* Could a donor materialize even before I launched my search? At that point, I wasn't mentally or emotionally prepared for a donor to arrive. John is a relative I hadn't seen in years. Our previous interactions were restricted to family functions—holiday parties, weddings, and funerals. As we grew older, our parents, the linchpins of the extended family, passed away, and our contact ceased. Individuals went their separate ways. But his offer came with some authority. His only sister, Cathy Jorgensen, had donated a kidney to my aunt, Marge Bencivenga, fifteen years earlier. I knew generosity was abundant in his family.

John was effusive and committed, and I was struck by his enthusiasm and willingness. As we talked, one caveat emerged—he has chronic fatigue syndrome. His primary care doctor told him his condition wouldn't prevent giving me a kidney. He agreed to call my donor nurse, Kathy Davis, at UChicago's Transplant Center. I was cautiously optimistic but still reeling at the suddenness of his offer. *Am I going to cross the goal line after a few weeks?* Emotionally, the door was ajar. A quick solution seemed unlikely after all the stories I'd heard about finding a donor. But with Audrey's support, I got on board. *It's possible,* I mused, *maybe, just maybe . . .*

Motivated and excited by John's eagerness to get things going at UChicago's Transplant Center, I gave him instructions on how to start the process. He phoned Kathy Davis the following day. By that evening, he'd been eliminated. Hope was extinguished as swiftly as it had arrived. I was worried about his preexisting condition, but what derailed his effort was being treated for high blood pressure—a deal breaker for donors. The roller-coaster ride had begun.

When I started to head in one direction, an unanticipated issue would emerge somewhere else, demanding a new course. This process of misdirection or reversal became indicative of my search. Taking John's call that evening, various feelings emerged: disappointment, anxiety, a sense of inevitability, and sadness. This array of emotions became familiar in the months that followed. It wouldn't be the last time I thought I had a donor only to have the circumstance change abruptly. When that happened, a protective emotional mechanism automatically kicked in. It was a shielding measure I expressed only to Audrey or myself: *So it goes* . . . (I'm borrowing that expression from Kurt Vonnegut's *Slaughterhouse-Five*). I empathized with John, who was truly disappointed about not being able to donate. John's reaction sensitized me to the emotional toll donors experience when they offer a gift of such magnitude and it's rejected. The potential donor's altruism, zeal, and commitment can be quickly dashed, resulting in a deep sense of loss and disappointment.

Sharon had described how her donor, Paul May, was transformed by donating a kidney. Initially, I was unable to fully comprehend what she said. I was too new to the game, and my perspective was too narrow. John's offer and his rejection gave me a frame of reference— and the lightbulb glowed. I grasped, not just intellectually but emotionally, how profound donating was to the giver. At first look, it appears as if the recipient is the only beneficiary of a gift. But as I heard from Sharon and witnessed in my story, the donor can also experience a deep, hidden, even transformative benefit from sharing such a monumental gift.

Donating an organ is on a short list of comparably heroic and altruistic acts: running into a burning building to save someone, perhaps, or a Medal of Honor winner's lifesaving act. But what distinguishes the act of giving an organ is that it is done quietly, over time, and behind the scenes. It requires a progressive commitment and a humility that truly puts another human being first. Saving another person through organ donation is an elongated commitment that takes the giver down a gauntlet of medical testing; it's not a single heroic gesture. Organ donation requires time and perseverance, facets of the process that are often overlooked but are another part of what distinguishes donors.

Even though I hadn't located a donor, the next weeks were filled with a series of medical tests. Extensive blood labs, an ultrasound to check the number and size of the cysts on my kidneys, an electrocardiogram (ECG), stress tests, and an MRI were all completed as a prerequisite for official admission to the transplant program. Acceptance marked a transition out of limbo into the more defined, but still strange, murky, and confusing world of hospitals and medicine.

While waiting to locate a donor, I realized my go-to strategies of avoidance, denial, and magical thinking were now completely useless. That triumvirate had been an indispensable ally in my earlier fight for survival, but now I needed to let it go. A number of psychological research studies report short-term avoidance and denial allow you to cope with the gravity of the bigger, scarier reality in your life. Denial allowed me to deflect, at least for a while, the blows and assaults that abrasively accompany a degenerative disease. They helped me survive moment to moment and endure over time. Life was radically different for me now, though, and I discovered that the most functional strategy was direct engagement.

One direct-engagement effort I continued was exercise, a practice I'd followed all my adult life. In fact, wellness was so important to me that it was the topic of my doctoral dissertation. Consequently, even with my new reality of end-stage renal disease (ESRD), I made every effort to stay healthy. Exercise gave me the sense of doing something positive and constructive for myself. It empowered me. The thought of idly waiting for my kidneys to completely fail was depressing and potentially emotionally crippling. With this attitude in mind, and as part of the process to have a kidney transplant, I would have to get a stress test to assess my cardiovascular condition and determine if I could withstand the surgery. My goal that spring was to be able to last an hour on the elliptical trainer at the gym before I took my stress test on a treadmill. Summoning Zeus-like energy and with great effort I accomplished my objective. Passing that stress test was a personal triumph. I celebrated as if I had climbed Everest or swum the English Channel. As the months passed and my disease worsened, my stamina waned. My March accomplishments had long faded by August and September.

While waiting for things to unfold with Al (his offer was put on hold because of his age and the decision to attempt to get a family member's kidney) and John's initial offers to donate, Roseann and I started talking about her giving me a kidney. During our conversations and emails, she reminded me that she'd offered me a kidney twenty years earlier. I'd long forgotten her proposition and generosity. Now her renewed offer was in play, and it was the center of my universe. Emails flew back and forth. She wrote:

> My blood type is O positive, yes, the universal donor. I'll get tested if your doctors agree. I'm not sure I'm qualified, however, because of Rob's hepatitis C, as no one in our house is allowed to donate blood because we live with him. Then there's the cancer thing, but that's over.

When I replied that I didn't want to pressure her, she wrote:

> No pressure, I always said I'd see if I could donate if you got to this point. Really, we Baldaufs aren't easy to pressure into anything . . . ☺

My sister had decisively thrown her kidney in the ring and was now the leading contender to donate. I was ecstatic . . . and optimistic.

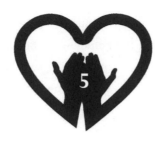

KIDNEY HUNTING

There are few perfect survivors. . . . There are many, though, who
flail around at first, then get their minds right, and live.

—LAURENCE GONZALES, *DEEP SURVIVAL*

The tests to assess the viability of my having kidney transplant surgery were ongoing. In addition to the treadmill stress test, they included a CAT scan, extensive blood labs (twenty-one vials were taken), an ECG, and an ultrasound. I must have done well overall because I was accepted as a good candidate for surgery, as healthy enough to receive someone else's kidney. It seemed a bit ironic to be "healthy" enough to get a transplant. My official acceptance was a welcome relief and "green lighted" my search. The first obstacle—testing—was effectively maneuvered. Full speed ahead. We had another reason to celebrate.

Admission into the transplant program meant I was placed on a national registry to receive a cadaver kidney. When monthly blood labs were taken, a vial was sent to Gift of Hope Organ & Tissue Donor Network, a national organization that maintains a database to track individuals who agree to be donors upon their deaths. Although relatively new, this group was a godsend to countless people in need of a kidney. If a kidney became available that "perfectly" matched my blood and tissue type, I would be pushed to the top of the list and given the opportunity to accept the kidney. The phrase "I'm on a waiting list for a kidney" (or heart, liver, or other organ) generally refers to this process. Traditionally, and regrettably, unless the available kidney is a "perfect match," a person can spend anywhere from three to five years on one of these lists.

Although the availability of organs has increased because of technology, volunteer donor designations on driver's licenses, and Gift of Hope and other registries, the wait time for organs is a national crisis. Many European countries (around twenty-five) are light years ahead of the United States. Instead of asking citizens to donate their organs in the event of an accident, people are automatically considered donors and an individual must opt out by actively requesting to *not* be on the list. Additionally, all emergency and medical personnel are alerted when an organ transplant is possible, resulting in a more efficient and effective organ transfer system.

It was comforting to know there was some support for my search, though, even if the United States needs to work on some improvements. Consumed by wondering where a kidney would come from, I appreciated in a new way the people who checked the donation box on their driver's license application. People willing to donate their organs are special. Donors, living or dead, are unsung heroes who give people like me the chance to reclaim our lives. Because someone somewhere casually checked that box on a routine application, another person in dire need of a transplant could get lucky. (My brother Tom received his kidney from a person in a fatal motorcycle accident.) Still, I wanted donor database to be the backup plan. Audrey and I remained dedicated to finding a living donor.

A living donor was the best option because the life expectancy of the kidney and its ability to function after transplant are optimized. In a living-donor transplant, the donor and I would be in connected operating rooms and prepared almost simultaneously. When the kidney was harvested, the surgeon would literally carry the kidney into the operating room where I was waiting. Then the surgeon would implant the kidney into my body. How amazing is that? A living miracle. When my wonderful surgeon, Dr. Yolanda Becker, described this process during my pre-op visit a week before my surgery, she was beaming and filled with glee. Hearing that she liked to take the kidney in her hands so that she could feel the life in it gave us goose bumps. (The hospital preferred she place it in a sterile bowl for donor-to-recipient transport, which she did.) The process sounded so astonishing, you almost *wanted* to have a kidney transplant. It was heartening that my surgeon reveled in her work. Her palpable enthusiasm was contagious.

Finding a suitable, healthy donor was my primary focus for the next seven months. Little did I know what a roller-coaster ride it would be. The stress and exhaustion was accompanied by a growing worry that I might fail. For a while, it seemed as if the odds were against us. But it also was motivating. Irrepressible optimism found its way back to us after the setbacks we experienced.

Audrey wrote the family the following email:

> Yesterday we spent several hours with the Transplant Team at UChicago (nephrologist, surgeon, nurse, social worker). We couldn't be more impressed with their empathy, professionalism, knowledge, and efficiency. As someone in the medical profession, I'm a pretty tough critic.
>
> We found out Greg's blood type is O, so we need someone who is O (negative or positive doesn't matter) to be willing to donate a kidney. They want the donor to be under sixty years old. They can facilitate this being done in six weeks once we have a donor. He's also on the national list for a cadaver donor; living donors are much better for the recipient, so we're hoping that will work out.
>
> Of course, we had hoped this day would never come, but since it has, I believe we've come to

peace with it and are ready to move to the next step.
We hope this can happen by May or June because
he has lots of dancing to do at Emily's wedding on
October 1.

Much love, Audrey

Audrey and I frequently discussed the most likely candidates among
our family and friends. *Who will step forward? Who could be a blood and
tissue match? How do you ask another person for a body part?* These were
questions we pondered, morning and night. In the course of a day
or week we would move between hope, optimism, fear, anxiety,
desperation, and loneliness—some of them simultaneously. The
sober reality of it all was clear during or after our conversations
even though life had taken on a surreal quality. My perceptions were
distorted. Frequently I slipped into dysfunctional, perseverating
thoughts, which adversely affected my thinking and my ability to
perform routine daily activities.

Searching for a kidney was a twofold process. First, find a generous
person who's willing to donate, and, second, get the person tested to
determine if he or she is physically able to donate and have the surgery.
Finding potential donors was unnerving, but waiting to see if they
qualified was worse. The final outcome would likely determine my
future, including quality of life, level of function or disability, and the
potential necessity of ongoing dialysis. Never having been in a situation
like this, the tidal pull of potential failure threatened a despair and
numbness I feared could result in mental and emotional paralysis. I
never froze entirely; I consciously and vehemently resisted it. I found
the support to press forward. But the anxiety was considerable, and
I did experience depression. I understand now how a person in this
situation can slip, get stuck, or even give up. The heaviness of the
situation caught up with me, and sometimes I felt overcome with

lethargy. As my bodied weakened, so did my spirit at times. I was fortunate these moods were short-lived.

Audrey and our family and friends were available when things were at their most exasperating. Any one of them could redirect me to a healthier mind-set via their optimism, humor, or kindness. My children's natural buoyancy was contagious. They helped me help myself. I doubt I would have persisted alone or unsupported. If people who loved me believed and trusted, then so would I. I stayed the course, albeit with a misstep or two . . . or three. Persistence and perseverance were essential. Initially I thought my situation was only about my physical condition and the ensuing medical intervention. But what started as a medical and physical threat and potential tragedy evolved into so much more: living.

Still focusing on my extended family, I was unsure of who else might be able to donate a kidney. Two of my second cousins, Cathy Jorgensen and Paul May, had done so for Aunt Marge fifteen years earlier and my cousin Sharon Gitzen about twelve years earlier, respectively. Who was left? Who was young enough and had a healthy kidney? Some of the younger Baldaufs (including my brother Tom's children—Tom, Mike, Donna, Jonn, and Eric) who were possible donors might have to save their kidney for a sibling. In fact, Tom's second son, Mike, lovingly offered, but I couldn't in good conscience move forward with him. Realistically, Mike needed to save that kidney for one of his siblings to have in the future.

Judging by her recent emails and our long-standing relationship, the most likely candidate was still my sister, Roseann. She was five years younger than me and in good health. Jerry, seven years my senior, was an unlikely candidate because of his age and the fears about his health that he'd discussed in recent emails. Dr. Nash told me that everyone began losing kidney function at around forty years of age, approximately 1 percent a year. Having already lost kidney function, people over sixty aren't ideal candidates. For an older donor, losing a kidney is potentially harmful, in case he or she has a serious kidney-related health issue. And it wouldn't be optimal for me to go through a transplant for a kidney with already decreased functioning. Only if no other options were open and I was at death's door would an older kidney come into play.

As my attention turned to my sister, Uncle Bill and Aunt Irene sent out an email to even more family members: "Bill's nephew, Greg Baldauf, needs a kidney transplant due to his kidneys failing from PKD (polycystic kidney disease)." Bill and Irene were the patriarch and matriarch of the extended Baldauf family and the relatives to whom I was closest over the years. At that time, Bill was eighty-five and had PKD. He was my father's youngest brother, and the last surviving member of his generation. Uncle Bill was my role model for living well with PKD. I had figured if he made it to his mideighties without dialysis or a transplant, so could I. As a boy, he was my favorite uncle—always magically pulling quarters out of my ears when he visited. Now the equivalent to the magic quarter was surviving without a transplant.

Sadly, Bill had suffered the losses of three siblings: Carl from complications due to PKD; my father, George, who had the disease but died from other causes; and Marge, less than two years after her transplant. No fifty-fifty genetic split among their generation—all four siblings who survived to adulthood had PKD. (Their oldest sibling, Henry, died as a child of pneumonia. It's unknown if Henry also had PKD.) Uncle Bill had to witness, repeatedly, how devastating PKD can be. There's an added emotional burden for the one who survives. The survivor is haunted by the losses and knows this could be his fate as well. Consequently, my uncle and aunt were diligent observers of PKD in our family. When I reached the point of needing a transplant, they responded with lightning speed, offering love, help, and support.

* * * * *

The process of donating a kidney is paradoxically simple and complex. In my case, a potential donor would call the Transplant Clinic and speak to Kathy Davis—nurse, gatekeeper, and protector of a possible donor. She was caring and professional, but also stern, tough, and thorough. An intimidating presence, Kathy loomed large in the clinic. UChicago is the epicenter for the study of medical ethics, so it's no surprise they have a rigorous protocol in place to keep donors safe and free of coercion, and donors and recipients separate. The hospital didn't want me or any other recipient to influence a possible donor—overtly or covertly. The designated donor section of the clinic adhered to these standards religiously. Unquestionably this was an excellent practice, but I was taken aback at how passionately this procedure was followed. Not intending to undermine it, we managed to sidestep the process slightly because my potential donors informed us of their progress throughout the process.

My insurance covered the potential donor's expenses, and only one candidate could be processed at a time, which meant it wasn't possible to work from a list to determine the best candidate. With that said, becoming a donor was essentially a three-step process. Step one: Kathy Davis screened the potential donor via a phone interview to determine if he or she was eligible to proceed. Step two: If the initial medical screening was successful, blood labs were ordered for the candidate to discover if the blood type was compatible and to determine any tissue matches. Although there are apparently close to a hundred different tissues in the body in play related to compatibility, evaluations for kidney matches focus on six tissue types. Step three: If the donor was compatible, he or she was required to visit the UChicago hospital for extensive medical testing.

One of my strongest motivations for writing this book emerged from the mystery surrounding people who donate their organs or even consider doing so. The altruism and unselfishness of donors inspires me. I was captivated by donors' willingness to undertake a task of this nature, and I wanted to understand it. Their altruism is complex, and their motivation for donating an organ may not even be entirely known to them. Their deeply personal reasons may be elusive or unconscious. Giving someone an organ might be one of those unexplainable miracles that emerge from the very best part of what it means to be human. Giving an organ to restore another's life is an amazing and loving act. One way to view organ donation is that it helps counterbalance negative forces and hatefulness in the world. Donating celebrates the power of the human spirit to heal oneself and others. Altruism of this magnitude is extremely difficult to describe or comprehend—and being the beneficiary of such immense generosity is no less intricate. When I studied with the Andean shamans in Peru, my teacher had a saying: "It cannot be taught; it can only be experienced." These words resonate with what transpires between a donor and recipient. The experience reveals the deeper meaning of giving and receiving, largely at an unspoken level.

To illustrate even further the mysterious nature of what was happening as my search started, a potential donor, a stranger in Ohio, *found me.* My daughter Emily had recently moved to Chagrin Falls, Ohio, with her then-boyfriend, Terry Parmelee, and shortly after, they got engaged. As my saga unfolded, Emily mentioned my need for a kidney to her future father-in-law, who then retold it to a young friend of his, Bret Williams. Astonishingly, Bret said he would give me a kidney. His quick, unflinching response seemed strange and, to be totally honest, I was somewhat suspicious. Foolishly, by not engaging him at the time, I essentially turned him down. Can you believe it?

But his offer baffled me. Even though I was consumed with finding a kidney, I was ill-prepared to deal with actually getting one. *Why*, I wondered, *would some twenty-seven-year-old stranger from Ohio want to give an old guy like me a kidney?* I asked Terry to extend my thanks to Bret, but tell him my sister was likely going to donate. Trying to be polite, I said, "If things don't work out with Roseann, I'll get back to him."

At the time, I believed family members made better donors, which isn't always true even though immediate family members, particularly siblings, have a greater chance of more genetic tissue matches.

Still at the beginning of my search, my ignorance and naiveté were increasingly evident. In retrospect, my foolish, knee-jerk decision to reject Bret's offer could have easily turned out to be a disaster. As my journey continued, I began to wonder if I wasn't really in charge of what was happening or what the results were going to be. The emerging process far exceeded my control, but it seemed guided by more than just blind, dumb luck. Being conscious and able to act when the opportunity presented itself was required. Unbeknownst to me at the time, Bret, who had entered my life randomly, would become an integral part of my journey within a matter of months.

As my search progressed, I discovered that the kind of unhesitating response Bret displayed was how individuals willing to donate an organ frequently reacted. Of the eight people who offered me a kidney—one of whom was a complete stranger I met by chance at a lunch with work friends—most did so in an unflinching, matter-of-fact, and immediate fashion. The manner of their response, so emphatic and assured, led me to suppose humans must have a gene for altruism. A response of this seriousness and significance had to come from somewhere in their human nature or constitution. Their willingness to give had to have previously existed in their psyche.

On March 1, 2011, wanting to enlist as many people in the search as possible, I sent the following email:

> Dear family and friends,
>
> As many of you know (apologies to anyone I haven't yet talked to personally about this), my lifelong struggle with polycystic kidney disease (PKD) worsened last December. I'm now working with the UChicago Kidney Transplant Team to get a living donor kidney as soon as possible. My current kidney function is down to approximately 15 percent. As

I continue to lose kidney function in the coming months, I run the risk of having to go on dialysis, something my doctors and I both hope to avoid. I've been told that for each year a patient is on dialysis; his life expectancy drops 5 to 10 percent. Therefore, my goal is to get a transplant before dialysis is required.

My sister Roseann has incredibly and generously offered to donate one of her kidneys and is currently undergoing the review process to see if she's eligible. Because she has an O blood type (a blood match decreases the chance of rejection) and because we share parents, she provides the best chance for the recommended six tissue matches. The more matches, the better my chance of keeping the kidney longer.

In general, odds are higher for matches with family members.

Because my insurance covers the cost of the medical assessment for the donor, the protocol at UChicago is to work with one donor at a time.

All that said, there's no guarantee these initial donor possibilities will work out. The situation requires that I put the word out to as many people as possible in order to discover how many people are willing to consider donating a kidney.

Believe me when I say this is the most humbling thing I've ever had to do. The surreal task of asking someone for a body part to sustain my life is incredibly difficult to even describe. But ask I must.

There are two options for anyone willing to consider donating a kidney: 1) If you're a blood match (type O), you could donate a kidney directly to me. 2) If you aren't a blood match, but would still consider donating, it would be possible to participate in the National Kidney Registry. In that case, you give a kidney to someone else, allowing me to get a kidney that matches my blood type and tissues from someone else in the registry.

If you were to consider being a donor, here are some things to think about:

- Donors should be in excellent health
- Preferably under sixty years of age
- Have blood type O (in the case of option 1)
- Absence of any current cancer, high blood pressure, or diabetes (a past cancer isn't necessarily a deal breaker)
- The donor's medical costs are paid by my insurance

There are no complications (other than recovery from laparoscopic surgery) or correlations with other medical problems in the future for the donor (however, you might have to give up kickboxing.)

If you're interested, know someone who might be interested, or would like more information, please contact me or Audrey. We'll do our best to answer any additional questions—but, more importantly, we'll refer you to the nurse in charge of assessing potential donors.

There's no way I'll ever be able to thank you enough for even considering this request, but please know I'll always hold you in my heart.

I understand that not everyone is willing or able to be a living donor. However, please feel free to pass on my request to anyone you think might consider it.

Audrey, the kids, and I trust this process will ultimately prove successful. No doubt it will be an interesting journey (and, for me, an adventure of a lifetime). Thank you for participating in it with us. Thank you for listening.

Sincerely, Greg

The ensuing responses were remarkable and disorienting. More people offered to give me a kidney. For various reasons—age, health, and blood type—they couldn't do so. But the very act of offering astonished me. I sobbed in my office as I read their replies.

Susan Eriksen had already thought it over and emailed, "Offering to participate in the 'kidney-swap-o-rama.'"

Wendy Kopald wrote, "I can understand how humbling this must feel, and I am so glad you asked this community of people who care so much about you to consider this. . . . It is a lot to think about. As you hold us in your heart, I hold you in mine. I too feel a deep sense that this will work out for you. . . . I will think about this. I will pass this on and I send you so much love."

My loving friend from Florida, Randy Zatrock, replied, "Sign me up. I'm not sure I qualify (sixty-four years of age and A+ blood), but if you or the donor network want me, I'll do it."

Their genuineness had a profound effect on my emotional well-being. This new chorus of love and support was a gift that went straight to my heart. Even though my body was slowly deteriorating, emotionally and spiritually I was infused with an unconditional love I'd never before experienced. I gradually absorbed this goodness into my heart. I never truly felt alone or adrift because of the love my friends and family demonstrated. Their support sustained me throughout the search and long after the surgery and my recovery were complete.

With my optimism supercharged, I turned my attention to my sister being my donor and . . . my hero.

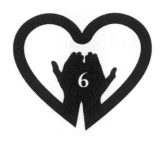

STEPPING UP, STEPPING OUT, STEPPING IN

Gratitude, humility, wonder, imagination, and cold, logical determination: those are the survivor's tools of mind.

—Laurence Gonzales, *Deep Survival*

Roseann and I love each other. She is the youngest child in our family and the daughter my mother always wanted. Being the "baby girl" with three older brothers, she learned to survive and thrive in a testosterone-driven, patriarchal German-Polish family with a hypercritical mother. We both eventually became closer with our father: me, as I worked in his butcher shop from age eleven into my college years, and Roseann, as the youngest who was around him more after he mellowed in retirement, becoming kinder and less intense. Sharing a positive relationship with our father strengthened my relationship with Roseann in our adult years, as did becoming our parents' caretakers as they aged. Our connection was also reinforced by living just fifty miles apart.

Even though I tricked her into making peanut butter and jelly sandwiches for me for a penny when she was five years old, she was still willing to give me a kidney when she was fifty-five. One striking aspect of her offer was that she was so matter-of-fact about it. When I worked up the courage to discuss it with her directly, she appropriately said she needed to discuss it with her husband, Rob Shales, and two teenage children, Robbie and Ricky. They weighed in: "You have to do it; he's your brother." Within a day's time, I had a donor and, with luck, a kidney. The pall of worry that had filled my every waking hour for months lifted with her consent.

Our conversation that day in early February when she agreed and confirmed her commitment was sweet and tender. Tearing up as I expressed my appreciation, she responded, "You really didn't think I wouldn't give you a kidney, did you?" Discussing the process of being a donor and casually joking and laughing, we plodded through the details. I knew Roseann, a dynamo and juggernaut, would be on top of getting connected to the Transplant Clinic. As a result of her enthusiasm and effectiveness, I joked we could possibly do the transplant the next day. Our relaxed exchange that day was typical of how we interacted . . . except for the fact I was in renal failure.

I thought there were two potential problems with my sister giving me a kidney. She had been diagnosed with uterine cancer three years earlier, and even though the intervening procedure was successful, the cancer's potential return could be a problem. The second issue was that her husband, Rob, a fireman and a onetime paramedic, contracted hepatitis C on the job and was treated for it a few years earlier. Consequently, living with him put her at risk of contracting hep C. Both concerns registered with me, but I was optimistic. I believed Roseann would be screened, tested, and cleared. I'd get her kidney and live happily ever after. I wanted so badly to be saved that I was unrealistic about how the process of getting a kidney unfolds. She was going to be my hero, and I told her so. There was a not-so-subtle seduction in this kind of thinking. I imagined the headline would read: SISTER GIVES

BROTHER A KIDNEY; SAVES HIS LIFE. Magical thinking is a powerful way—and a necessary one, to a point—to keep the demons at bay.

Roseann and Jerry had been spared the PKD chromosome. Ironically, her good fortune was to be mine now too. I was genuinely never angry that I had PKD while two of my siblings didn't. Nor did I blame my father for passing it on to me. Having a degenerative disease like PKD forms a peculiar bond with other family members who share the experience. The culture of our extended family reflects a silent sensitivity to those with PKD. After Tom died, my siblings discussed my condition between them, but rarely directly to me because they worried it would upset me. Jerry and Roseann were keeping a silent vigil regarding my health. Now their concern was activated.

Audrey was overjoyed and teary when we discussed Roseann's offer. We breathed a sigh of relief. I emailed the kids with the good news, calling later that night to discuss it further. When a family is starving for good news, everyone grabs it when it arrives. We attempted to be realistic. We knew doubt and fear would return, but we indulged ourselves in the hopeful scenario. We even precariously speculated about the best time for the surgery. Roseann wanted it in April because Rob was scheduled to have another treatment for his hepatitis C. We thought May was best so I could complete my semester at the college. We were getting ahead of ourselves, but it was exciting to discuss the possibilities. Later, when problems arose and the roller-coaster ride became too much to handle, we learned to temper our exuberance.

My sister flew through the initial screening and started the testing. I got daily reports on what was happening. One snag emerged during her testing. She described it in an email:

> Here's where I am . . . . Waiting for approval from
> Greg's insurance for cross-matching and blood
> tests. I was going to have blood samples drawn on
> Monday but insurance approval isn't yet confirmed
> and the test for one of the three things needed is
> over $2,000. So hopefully will be able to go later

next week. I am O positive, and hopefully my 2008
uterine cancer won't be a problem. I know it is
gone, just need pathology to show that to be true.
This is just the beginning, but my gut tells me I'll
match. We'll see if that proves to be true.

The high-speed train I was riding was derailed by the bureaucracies
of the insurance company and the hospital. What initially looked
like a minor and temporary pause turned into a month-long fiasco.
There was confusion about Roseann's medical costs being covered.
My fragile confidence crumbled, and emotionally I went from sixty to
zero in seconds. My express train stopped and didn't restart again for
almost thirty days.

Initially, learning that my health insurance would cover the would-
be donor's costs had been a pleasant surprise. That coverage eliminated
burdensome financial issues around getting a donor. Money wouldn't
be the reason I succeeded or failed to get a kidney. But now insurance
coverage transformed into another problem to be solved. With the
help of the insurance specialist at the college, Beth Taylor, another
everyday hero, it was clear from reading the policy that any donor
would have their medical expenses covered up to a million dollars.
Even their travel costs would be included, if needed. *So what the hell is
going on?* I wondered in frustration.

I made phone calls and talked to the insurance person at the
UChicago hospital and my primary caregiver's office. Finally, I
identified the problem. When the referral was made from my primary
care physician's office to UChicago's hospital, I was listed as a donor
rather than a recipient! This oversight by my doctor's office was the
ghost in the machine. Once identified, the two parties talked and the
problem was rectified. We were back on track. I was going to get that
kidney—or so I thought.

Navigating this insurance glitch taught me how important it is to be your own advocate, especially when the treatment is so complicated and the risks so profound. Had I not discovered the glitch and got the insurance person to talk to the hospital representative, I might still be waiting. What do individuals who are uneducated, have trouble reading, struggle with the language, or don't have a private medical specialist to consult with do? The breakdown left me feeling that at any time a patient can easily fall prey to either simple human error or the bureaucracy of medical insurance.

* * * * *

It was a tremendous credit to my sister that she involved me in her donor-evaluation process. Her inclusion allowed me to feel part of what is typically guarded or closed. Her updates kept me calm and, most importantly, optimistic. Here's an example of her savvy: on her first visit to the Transplant Clinic, she brought cookies to nurse Kathy Davis. Roseann was, after all, a saleswoman and businessperson. She knew how to make people comfortable and get them to immediately like her. *Way to go, Roseann,* I thought.

On April 4, prior to even meeting Kathy Davis, Roseann sent an email to me and Audrey detailing what a donor had to get through:

> I think the timing has to do with the tests. It must take time for the cross match to see if antibodies develop. She (Kathy Davis) didn't indicate what's next. From what I gather online, there are twelve steps to get through to donate. I also filled out a questionnaire with medical history and doctor info. She said earlier that they wanted the pathology reports on the uterine cancer, so I included info for the doctor. I think the last week of May should work. I have trips for work through the third week.

Here are the steps I found on kidney.org/transplantation:

1. Financial/insurance consult

2. Immunological tests (that's what the blood was for now)

3. Other labs for systems functions and screens for disease

4. EKG for heart function

5. Medical history and physical

6. Psychiatric evaluation

7. Gynecological exam and mammogram

8. Kidney function test

9. Possibly intravenous pyelography and X-rays to identify kidney structure

10. Helical CAT scan to evaluate internal kidney structure and maybe X-rays

11. Renal arteriogram (maybe) if they need more info after the helical CAT scan

12. All results to transplant team (surgeons, counselors, nurses, social workers, etc.) to determine suitable candidate

Even being familiar with Roseann's matter-of-fact attitude, her email blew us away. After reading the detailed list of what was involved medically for the donor to give a kidney, I cried. I knew donating was extensive and demanding; but after actually reading the list, I thought anyone willing to do this was crazy or a saint. Previously, Audrey and I had thought her attitude toward giving me a kidney was as if she were going to the dentist to have her teeth cleaned—the task was slightly unpleasant, a bit time-consuming, but no big deal. But living donors have to run a gauntlet even before an organ is harvested and given to another human being. The sacrifice and commitment required grabbed my heart and squeezed it.

Roseann was incredibly committed, thorough, and dedicated. She was also remarkably optimistic and nonchalant. Her approach to the demanding medical maze came across as if she were completing a grocery list. She derived immense satisfaction from checking off the endless items required of her. My sister is a hero—as are all living donors and those who attempt to donate.

On April 12, before meeting with Kathy Davis and having only contacted her over the phone for preliminary tests, Roseann emailed and concluded with: "Hurdle #1 done . . . . This just takes patience!" Her note was a powerful reminder that my path was inherently fraught with difficulties, but they could be overcome. A change in my attitude could reframe a threatening problem into a challenge. This emerging perspective created more energy, informed my consciousness, and enlightened my attitude to the whole process. This episode of my life was occurring on multiple levels: on the physical level, of course, but also on emotional and spiritual dimensions. What was unfolding was inspiring and filled with gifts and opportunities to live more fully. Even though the quality of my life hung in the balance, my quest for a donor would get resolved one way or another.

I realized the outcome of my physical predicament wasn't the only experience I was having. The *process* itself was. Of course, I wanted a healthy and happy resolution. But I also knew that the ending to my story was ultimately out of my control. I started being more aware of the present moment and tried to stay in it. My awareness of *living* increased exponentially. With few exceptions in my very ordinary life, an in-the-moment experience was rare. What was currently happening was rich, uncertain, and even life threatening, but it was unmatched in intensity. I was fully conscious of living. It was ironic that this experience of fullness was brought about by the threat of severe decline or death.

With the insurance issue eliminated, Roseann and I seriously pursued possible surgery dates. She intended to have a conversation with Kathy Davis about timing. The hospital staff started to discuss possible dates for surgery as early as June. We were almost there. A sense of relief grew in me. Audrey felt it too, and the kids weren't far behind. April started with a great deal of momentum. The transplant was going to happen, right? I was so optimistic that on April 13 I sent out an email with the subject line "Greg's Transplant—Hallelujah!":

> Dear family and friends,
>
> I received some wonderful, spectacular, and awesome news yesterday from my sister Roseann. She's a blood and tissue match and can be a living donor! Hallelujah.
>
> Although we're not entirely out of the woods yet (she has numerous tests to take before the final approval is given), the fact that we matched is a true cause for optimism and hope that this process will move forward with reasonable speed. As of yesterday, she was scheduled to test on May 11, 12, and 13. The transplant surgery could happen at the end of May or early June if everything checks out.
>
> It's very difficult to express exactly what this all means to me. Needless to say, I'm experiencing a tremendous amount of relief, wonderment, and humility. I'm truly overwhelmed by my good fortune. The tremendous vulnerability I've been experiencing is oddly still present. It's as if powerful forces are at work completely beyond my control. What a curious space to be in—no control at all and tremendous good fortune. I honestly don't know what would have happened if she wasn't a match. It's frightening to think about.
>
> Although not a serious devotee of karmic processes, I've often wondered in the past three months if my personal flaws and past mistakes might

not interfere with a donor becoming available. And
although I think this event is more a testament to my
sister's being good, generous, and gracious than it is
to my karmic merit, I'll accept that and run with it.
I'll do my best to graciously accept this little miracle.

Thank you again for your support, kindness, and
compassion over the past few months. I can't even
begin to tell you how helpful your love and care
has been for me and the family. I've struggled with
this situation and what it means, but I've never felt
alone. This awareness is a miracle in and of itself.

Please keep sending your kind thoughts and
words, prayers and meditations, and positive energy
to me. They're extremely healing and hopeful.

I'll keep you posted as this process unfolds. The
next announcement will hopefully include a date
for surgery.

With love and gratitude, Greg

The responses invigorated us. It felt like I heard from everyone in
my life and then some: family members, former students, friends,
colleagues, fellow men's group participants, friends with whom I'd
studied Andean shamanic ways, and even acquaintances. All offered
love, wisdom, support, and blessings. I was buoyant, as if I were actually
being lifted up and carried. No matter the outcome, I was being given
a gift beyond my wildest imagination—unconditional love.

My cousin Sharon, kidney recipient and mentor to me in this
adventure, replied:

Glad to hear the great news. Yes, each step is a miracle
in itself. Your karmic life extends over time; thank
goodness it's not all in one lump. You are in the right
spot at the right time. It's exciting to see it all come
together for you. What a grand celebration. It's the

door and window thing: close, open. Life's lessons are
interesting. Sending you white light and prayers . . .

Phil Kirschbaum sent these words to me:

> I'm grateful to be in the feedback loop and to know
> about your progress toward a transplant. I'm not
> surprised but extremely pleased to hear about your
> sister's match as a donor. I'm envious of such a
> loving relationship with a sibling.
>
> You are such a treasure to us all, and this
> surgery and your healing will bring many blessings
> to those of us around you who are lucky enough to
> be your friend.

We were in a holding pattern until the middle of May, when Roseann
was scheduled for the lion's share of the medical tests. We waited
eagerly for the results, particularly the test for antibodies and antigens
in the blood. This test would determine if my body could accept the
new kidney. Our thoughts and hopes continued to turn to a date for
surgery. In hindsight, looking this far down the road was foolhardy.

I sent another email to my brother:

> As I email, my blood and Roseann's are being
> matched. It takes seven days to see if I've developed
> any antibodies, which could have happened when I
> was transfused because of that skiing accident in the
> mid-1980s. Ahh . . . the price of pleasure.
>
> With that said, I remain guardedly optimistic
> that she'll be a good-enough match. There's a
> 25 percent chance she'll be a perfect match and a
> 25 percent chance she won't match at all, which
> leaves an overall chance we'll match on some of
> the six tissues. A little Baldauf luck would be useful
> right now.
>
> When we get the go-ahead, there's about ten to
> twelve other medical procedures she'll have to go

through, but most of them are in preparation for surgery. There's even a psychological test she has to take.

We talked and we're looking at the last week in May for the transplant. Audrey and I even get a week in Florida before the event.

I'm assuming I'll be able to resume all normal activities, minus kickboxing. Audrey promises this fatigue and lack of energy I feel will vanish for the most part.

Our planned trip to Yosemite is doubtful right now. The postsurgical recovery is intense, e.g., daily trips to UChicago for examinations and tests. I guess the first month is the most critical in terms of my keeping the kidney. I can't imagine that I'll want to travel, but we'll see . . .

I'll keep you posted. Before this happened I was hoping to play Pebble Beach as a sixtieth birthday present from Aud. Saw Arnie and Jack tee off at Augusta this morning. Arnie always reminds me of you.

I'll let you know what happens next week.

All signs pointed to the surgery happening that spring. April flew by. In retrospect, I should have suspected things wouldn't be this easy or fast. I was caught up in the whirlwind of relief and wanting to be rescued. The progress being made reinforced our hopeful mood. Lost in the emotions of being so close to being saved, rational thought and caution were scarce.

The tide turned on May 5. Roseann sent Audrey and me an email with the subject line "Just Talked to Kathy Davis."

Greg and Aud,

My labs and panels came back OK. Protein a little elevated in twenty-four-hour urine. Chest X-ray normal. I have some gallstones, but I knew that.

All that said, there could be a deal breaker. My left kidney has a small benign angiomyolipoma—a small tumor of fat cells and muscle tissue. It grows very slowly and is something to watch when I have annual physicals. Because it involves the kidney, they could rule me out as a candidate. I still meet with the doctors next Wednesday and the donor panel will have reviewed it by then. I'm stunned by this info. I feel great and have been sure I could donate.

This thing usually grows very slowly. If they gave the kidney to Greg, it could respond to the immune suppressants and grow fast.

They'll have more info by next week and probably a decision. Aud, look into this and see what you can find out. I just talked with Kathy so I haven't Googled it yet.

Unexpectedly, the profound tenuousness of obtaining a donor emerged in a new way. A small tumor (two centimeters, or about the size of the top of a little finger) was discovered on one of Roseann's kidneys. Angiomyolipomas are benign fatty tumors that occur randomly in middle-aged women. Although slow growing and of no real danger to her, it was extremely problematic for me. The unexpected discovery of the tumor was a serious threat to our plan. When things "break bad," they do it convincingly. Our optimism came to a halt as fear replaced excitement. I did a 180-degree reversal, ruminating about the implications of the news.

Ironically, from the no-good-deed-goes-unpunished file, during the MRI to confirm the tumor, the machine broke down three times (it was blamed on the weather). She had to go to another machine in the research area to complete the test. This extended MRI experience was a challenge for my claustrophobic sister.

True to her nature, though, Roseann remained determined and optimistic. She was staunchly confident the tumor wouldn't prevent her from her appointed task. One doctor told her it would be best if she withdrew. I would do better with a healthier kidney. I was reminded that donating can become as essential to the donor as to the recipient, and that certainly appeared to be the case for my sister and me. A complex, intricate, and even mysterious relationship forms between the two people involved. It was impossible for me to not be moved by my sister's positive outlook and passion. Roseann would remain an option if things turned desperate. This current turn of fate, coupled with the complexity of the situation, was a warning sign. I recalled what the Transplant Clinic staff had said—the patient usually goes through four or five possible donors before they find one that works.

In the wake of my sister's news, I called Audrey. While discussing what had just happened, we recalled our initial commitment to be proactive. This sudden disruption was no time to alter our course. Keep pushing the boulder up the hill, regardless of the outcome. Don't panic or allow it to overcome you. Surrendering to fear or inertia at this point in time wasn't an option.

One upside to my kidneys failing later in my life was that I was the oldest in my family to get a transplant. My diseased, cyst-ridden kidneys had lasted a long time—a dubious distinction. The downside was that most of our friends and family were also sixty or beyond. Of people who had offered me a kidney, most were older. Sixty years of age is the cutoff point for donors. Knowing this wouldn't stop me from considering them if we thought my search would turn from months to years or my health worsened. Having a fallback position provided a modicum of relief. But at this point, we decided to keep our search within the family. The most likely candidate was my first cousin Ken Baldauf, Bill and Irene's son.

Emailing Ken rekindled my hopes as I tried to stay balanced on the tightrope. I needed a new hero. By contacting Ken, I was developing a connection with him as a potential donor, but continuing my involvement with my sister, tumor and all. Transitioning was delicate.

One benefit of my sister's medical issue was that Dr. Yolanda Becker became intricately involved with my situation. She was the director of UChicago's Kidney Transplant Department and relatively new at the university, having been there for approximately a year. She came from the transplant program at the University of Wisconsin Hospital, which performed the most kidney transplants per year in the country—almost five hundred. Without the slightest bit of ego or arrogance, she later told me she has probably done more transplants than anyone else in the country. Becker called to tell me she was devoting one of their Monday afternoon staff meetings to my particular case. The entire transplant team—nurses, surgeons, and nephrologists—were going to meet to discuss Roseann's condition. Thirteen doctors plus staff brainstormed ways to make my transplant happen. How cool was that? This plan reassured me about the quality of medical care I was receiving. My trust, already high, increased. With some of the smartest medical minds in country working on my case, a solution would be found, right?

Sadly, the result wasn't good. There were no positive aspects to using a donor with this complication. Dr. Becker had done a last-resort kidney transplant before with an angiomyolipoma located near the renal ducts. The kidney recipient was in and out of the hospital for a year as a result of postoperative bleeding. I didn't want to go through the ordeal of a transplant only to endure further medical complications with uncertain success. Becker's thinking was similar—because I was still relatively healthy and was only about six months into the search process, waiting was our best option. Disappointed, but understanding of the situation because of Becker's careful and rational explanation, I agreed. We moved on. My sister was relegated to only-in-an-emergency status.

What we thought was a slam dunk was a miss. My sister and I were deflated. Always a class act, Roseann graciously encouraged me to explore other options, most notably Ken. I knew I needed to move on to avoid succumbing to the stress of waiting.

On May 9, Roseann emailed:

> Greggie,
>
> Well, that's terrific (contacting Ken). I'll let you
> know what the kidney doc at UChicago has to say on
> Wednesday afternoon.
>
> I am certain this will all come together exactly as
> it is supposed to in the end.

Her last words were prophetic. We would still have to try and fail again
before it all came together.

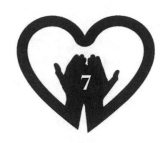

FROM THE ON-DECK CIRCLE TO THE BATTER'S BOX

*Do not dwell in the past, do not dream of the future, concentrate
the mind on the present moment.*

—Buddha

Ken was fifty years old and healthy. He was tested for PKD when he was a teenager and no cysts were found. His age, health, and status as a relative created a near-perfect donor scenario. The possibility of his giving me a kidney was first broached in March when his mother, my aunt Irene, spoke to him about donating. So Ken was already considering the possibility and waiting for the outcome of Roseann's tests. Given the complications with Roseann, Ken now vaulted to the top of my list.

Reeling from Roseann's essential elimination as a donor, I believed the only way to manage my anxiety was to contact Ken immediately. I needed to know if he was willing to pull the trigger and give me a kidney, so I emailed him.

> Minutes ago I found out Roseann has a tumor on
> one of her kidneys. It's not PKD or malignant, but it

will probably eliminate her as a donor for me. We'll get the final verdict on May 1. But obviously this is a sudden and unexpected turn for the worse.

I'm contacting you because your name has come up as a possible donor for me. And although I in no way want to put pressure on you to do this—it is an amazing thing for anyone to even consider—it would be helpful to me to know if you would, in fact, even consider doing this type of thing. The first thing I need to know is your blood type. I only match with an O.

If, for any reason, this isn't in the cards for you and me, that is, of course, OK—more than OK. I would completely understand. I'm at the point where I need to have a plan B, so I'm boldly putting this out there to you. Based on your response, I may need to broaden my request to anyone and everyone in order to get the process moving again.

I trust I'm being delicate and cautious enough with my asking. It's an extremely difficult thing to do, but I have a sense of urgency and need to move forward as best I can.

Please feel free to call if email seems a bit impersonal. Or you can give me your number, and I'll call you.

Thanks for hearing me out and even thinking about this.

Ken immediately replied:

I've been following your progress with this challenge and celebrated (albeit silently) with you upon the news of Roseann being a donor. I'm so sorry to hear of this recent turn of events. As you may have heard, I've been stymied trying to get my blood type. You'd think your doctor would know these things, but apparently not. Nor on a birth certificate, nor on

a wedding license or driver's license, nor at the lab
where I do my blood work. I'm embarrassed by how
much time has gone by since I started investigating
it. I was planning on going to a blood bank where
they would tell me my blood type when I got the
news about Roseann being a donor. Now with this
latest news, let me get into a blood bank or the
county health clinic or somewhere and get this
settled. I sure hope I'm able to help out with this.
I'm really glad you asked. Keep hanging in there,
and keep your hopes up.

He was kind and forthright and, most importantly, open to being a donor.
Hearing this from him was a tremendous relief. His honesty about my
situation gave me hope. After composing myself, I sent a response:

God bless you for being willing to have your blood
type checked. It's a testimony to your goodness
and grace.
   As soon as you know your blood type, please
let me know so we can, if necessary, move forward
on the application part of this. If not, I'll prepare
my mass appeal to the universe for a donor. ☹ I'll
keep you informed as things become clearer with
Roseann.
   I don't know how to even begin to thank you,
Ken, for considering this. It brought tears to my eyes
this morning and gives me reason to hope. Anyone
in my position would tell you that people like you
are very, very special people.

Consistent with what characterized my experience so far, the situation
and my emotions were again altered suddenly and dramatically. Up
and down the kidney-search roller coaster I went. Within a five-day
span, I was back in the game. One door closed, another opened.

Ken was soft-spoken, gentle, and thoughtful. His reserved manner fit the profile of a college teacher, author, and director of interdisciplinary computing at Florida State University. He'd been actively thinking about donating for months and was staying current about my situation via his mother and father and through emails with Roseann. My email inquiry pushed him from observer to participant, from the on-deck circle into the batter's box. I sensed he understood the gravity of my request. He graciously said he would discuss it with his wife and children and get back to me. I liked that my sister, and now Ken, thought a matter as serious as this needed to be processed with their spouses and families. That they each defaulted to that basic part of the decision first reveals the nature of their characters, and that instinct is probably entwined with their willingness to donate.

After discovering we share the same blood type and with his family's support, five days later, Ken confirmed he was ready and willing to participate. Tears (now frequent in my daily life) welled up in my eyes. Being the recipient of such goodness inspired awe. The matter-of-factness, simplicity, and humility of his decision and his ability to act were impressive. Based on his response, as well as my sister's, I thought these qualities must be present in any person willing to be an organ donor. There was an impressive grace about a donor's seemingly innate ability to be selfless. Good fortune and blessing walked next to me again. I kept thinking, *Holy shit and oh my God!*

Here's Ken's May 9 email to me:

> Hi, Greg,
>
> I have a voice mail in to Kathy Davis and expect that I'll be visiting a lab to send UChicago some blood.
>
> If it's OK with you, I'd like to keep my involvement in this a private matter between you, me, and our immediate families. I'm a little uncomfortable with the kind of attention a willing donor may receive. I hope you understand. Feel free to refer to me as the "candidate who prefers to

remain anonymous."You're a good man who I always respected and whose company I enjoy—as limited as that has been. I'll consider myself fortunate if I'm able to assist you with this. Feel free to phone any time.

By the way, I'm fortunate to enjoy very good health. If we're a match, I don't think you could find a better donor.

All the best!

Ken

After composing myself, I emailed him back: "WOW! I'm in shock. This is amazing news. You always looked like an O blood type to me. Again thank you so much. . . . Words can't do your generosity justice."

Ken began the process flawlessly and efficiently. With the blood type identified and Kathy Davis contacted, the process began. He passed the initial health screening and arranged to have the vials for the blood tests sent to him. His blood needed to be tested for antigens at UChicago's hospital. The tedious process of becoming a donor was jump-started because of his commitment and diligence. As you might expect from a person who worked in computing, Ken's attention to detail and his follow-up were exquisite. Momentum built as a result of his actions. Ken kept me, his parents, and my sister in the loop every step of the way.

Being kept apprised by both Roseann and Ken about the day-to-day status of their testing and their contact with Kathy Davis was heartening. Being included in the process remedied the worse aspect of looking for a donor—the not knowing. Ignorance leads to confusion and, ultimately, to fear. A partnership between the donor and recipient was atypical of the usual routine of donating at UChicago's hospital. The hospital's policy is to discuss medical information only with the patient—so in this case, only with the potential donors. I appreciated that Roseann and Ken were invested in keeping me updated on their side of the process.

Ken's assessment progressed normally. All the medical hoops were jumped through and requirements met. On May 23 Ken received insurance approval for the compatibility test of the antigens in our blood. He sent the sample immediately, reporting: "Six vials of my premium O+ blood are on their way to the UChicago Medical Center." The antigen test would determine whether either of our blood would reject the other. This test was critical to the transplant process, because I had some risk of having antigens after blood transfusions after a ski accident in the mid-1980s. The test revealed our blood was compatible. He could donate a kidney.

Interestingly, that decades-earlier ski accident—largely the result of me being a poor to mediocre skier—directly contributed to my current medical situation. For Veterans Day weekend in 1984, my dear friend Jim Bush and I went to Copper Mountain, a ski resort in Colorado. We arrived in time for the first big snow of the season. Despite being a novice, I managed to survive the whole day of skiing. By sunset, on my last run of the day, I "took air" and careened off a mogul, which knocked my elbow into my kidney and my kidney into my vertebra, rupturing a cyst and causing a massive internal bleed.

I wound up at the hospital in Vail after a stop at the clinic in Frisco, Colorado, and a treacherous ride in a mountain blizzard. For the entire ride I was in excruciating pain—the worst pain I'd ever experienced. I wound up losing two-thirds of my blood volume. Later I got six units of blood, some of it from people off the streets, including a Colorado State Patrol officer. Two fitful days later—the first night spent with Jim sleeping at the foot of my bed and the doctor conferring with Audrey on the phone about what to do, I was transported by ambulance to Colorado General in Denver. I was the highest-risk patient in intensive care. When the bleeding stopped, two large hematomas were surgically removed from my abdomen.

It took six months to recover physically and twelve months to recover emotionally. To complete my healing, I needed to return to the Colorado General Intensive Care Unit (ICU) a year later to make peace with what I'd experienced there and put some closure to my trauma. I asked permission to enter the isolated ICU room where I had spent the first few nights after arriving from the Vail hospital. Symbolically, returning to the ICU healthy and strong affirmed for me that I had recovered and could now move on. The trauma of my near-death experience was over. The visit allowed me to close the circle and feel whole once more.

This accident that damaged my kidney by opening the cysts, and the ensuing trauma, was likely the event that precipitated the degeneration of my kidney function. Though I wasn't aware of the phenomenon at the time, a common experience among PKD patients is that a physical trauma to the kidney triggers the beginning of renal failure and eventually a kidney transplant. I only learned about the occurrence of "precipitating events" about a year after my transplant surgery while conversing with a doctor from the Cleveland Clinic at a Walk for the Cure in Cleveland, Ohio.

Ken, with coaching from Audrey, scheduled a date to come for medical tests at the UChicago hospital. Following the protocol, Kathy Davis scheduled him in four weeks. Thinking this was an unnecessary wait if the transplant was going to happen in late July or August, we intervened. We wanted to move the process along as quickly as possible. With a bit of finagling, and some gentle nudging of Kathy Davis by Ken, the medical tests were moved up.

Roseann, fully on board with the transition from her to Ken, picked him up at O'Hare Airport and took him to the Transplant Clinic. As the donor procedure expert, who was better than my sister to walk Ken through the process and show him the ropes? Ken agreed. Because of her relationship with Kathy Davis, Roseann was an excellent conduit between the past and current situation, helping ease Ken into the strange world of becoming a donor.

After the first day of testing was completed, my two would-be donors arrived at our house in Evanston. Audrey and I thought a family dinner for all concerned was a good start, helping ease the stress Ken would go through. We invited Bill and Irene to join us, making it easier for Ken to see his parents without additional effort. We hoped to create the most relaxed situation possible in light of the seriousness of the overall situation. Dinner was wonderful, laughs flowed freely, and the tension eased. Everyone's spirits lifted, particularly mine.

Relaxing after dinner, I asked Ken how he felt about the possibility of giving me his kidney. His answer was captivating. "I always thought I would give someone in the family a kidney." He didn't know it would be me, but he knew from a relatively early age that—because of how PKD had affected various family members—he'd likely become a donor. The clarity of his premonition blew my mind. I never really considered the extended family members without PKD. My focus was on the family members with PKD and my own circumstances. Apparently, PKD or not, Ken and others were impacted by the disease too.

My perspective was self-centered and myopic. Ken's thinking was obviously farther reaching, and, honestly, more mature. I was enthralled by his attitude. The broader awareness our conversation inspired was another unexpected gift of my needing a kidney. It was another invitation to view my experience in a larger context. Renal failure, searching for a donor, and waiting for the impending transplant surgery were only parts of the totality of what was happening in our family.

Spending time with Ken and his father, who suffered from and worried about PKD, and his mother, also enlightened. Watching the three of them interact, I wondered, *What's it like for Bill and Irene to witness their son be tested to give me a kidney?* The juxtaposition of Bill and Irene wanting to help me, someone they cared for, but knowing their son would be at risk and need to live with one kidney was complex. There was a relatively small risk medically to donate a kidney, but abdominal surgery of any kind couldn't be minimized. Later that evening, moved by my hypnotic interest, I asked Bill and Irene about what they were thinking and the paradox I thought might exist for them. Their answer was what I expected: they wholeheartedly supported Ken giving me the kidney. I accepted their reply at face value. A sense of relief washed over me.

That evening with Ken, Bill, and Irene raised my consciousness and further committed me to the idea of writing this book about my experience set against the background of my extended family. I pledged to myself to help other families who struggle with PKD. I wanted to influence how they confront the renal failure and the transplant crisis.

I escorted Ken to the hospital the next two mornings. He underwent the series of required tests and met with the nephrologist and surgeon assigned to potential donors. Interestingly, the surgeon he consulted with was Dr. Becker. The tests, their results, and Ken's ensuing interviews with the doctors went smoothly and efficiently, flowing effortlessly because of his thoughtfulness, soundness, and ability to articulate what being a donor was all about for him. We left the hospital that second day feeling very optimistic. Would Ken become my donor? I grew more excited about this possibility with every passing hour. From a practical point of view, even though I was sad about my sister's frustrated efforts, I knew that getting a younger kidney would be beneficial for me. It was difficult not to be self-centered. My primary needs at the time were to be optimistic, keep moving forward, and extract the best from the situation.

That evening Audrey and I got to know Ken better. As we chatted over drinks and dinner, we found him extremely likable. By all indications, he's a good person who's kind, smart, and genuine. He impressed us with his integrity, his deep commitment to his work, and his love for his family. He lit up when he spoke of them, his books, and his work. Furthermore, he's the most soft-spoken member of the extended family, which is a striking contrast to most others in the group, who are often loud, boisterous, and outspoken. Talking with Ken that evening was a welcome relief to the commotion we'd lived for months. We envisioned him becoming my hero and my family's hero.

Ken joined the ranks of certain individuals able to donate with graciousness and selflessness. *Why do people do such a thing?* I kept wondering. It was humbling to be the beneficiary of this magnitude of compassion and generosity. I felt awe and gratitude. He was now my third hero to actively participate in my donor drama—first John, then Roseann, and now Ken (plus the others who had indicated their willingness to donate). The idea that I was participating in something that exceeded the physical plane was growing; this mysterious mind-boggling path was evolving into something far more transcendent.

Ken's last hospital visit consisted of an additional test and a meeting with Kathy Davis to summarize the experience and clarify where things stood. Though not obligated to attend this final meeting, he said, "Better to make the extra effort now than to have to come back later." We left thinking it would be smooth sailing from there on out. We even casually discussed dates for the transplant surgery. That afternoon, we rendezvoused with his parents and brother, who would then take him to the airport. Soon he'd be back in Florida with his family. Hugging good-bye we said, "See you soon." I immediately called Audrey with the good news. I was so close I could practically taste it.

We targeted late June or early July for surgery. We emailed regularly, particularly at times when Ken had been in touch with Kathy Davis. He diligently kept us up to date. We both wanted to get this thing over and done with. We were convinced it was going to happen. Bolstered by our optimism, we shared our enthusiasm with the kids and looked to the future.

Bad news arrived a few days later. The CAT scan results showed cysts on Ken's kidneys. The cysts were few in number, but enough to bring matters to a crashing halt. This news and its implications scared me to death. When we talked, he was apologetic and disappointed.

Imagine. He felt sorry for me. After all he'd done and gone through, he felt he'd let me down. Ken reported not being worried about his own health or what the cysts implied for his future. I took his words at face value, trusting it remained true for him. My interactions with my potential donors grew more and more intricate! I wasn't the only one facing consequences. Life is complex.

Bill and Irene emailed: "Our hearts go out to you, Greg and Audrey, as it must be devastating to have your hopes up high and then have not one but two great prospects rejected as donors. Let us know what we can do to help in the search for another donor. . . . We just wanted to let you know that we feel badly and are thinking of you." Irene and Bill's message summed up the moment eloquently and succinctly.

Ken wrote the next day: "I hope you are coping. Let me know what I can do to help." The empathy and compassion this family exhibited to us was incredible. His response also furthered my belief and awareness of how emotionally involved the donor becomes in this process.

With Ken eliminated, I was near panic. I was fresh out of family members who would or could donate. The next step, most likely, was a widespread SOS to everyone and anyone I'd ever met. I was at the point of emailing friends, former students, everyone at the college where I worked, and everyone at the hospital where Audrey worked. This option was extremely intimidating and discouraging. My circumstances were rapidly spinning out of control (although I realized *control* was but a euphemism). I felt nauseated. I moved one step closer to dialysis. My emotions were raw and I was irrational in retrospect. I was inundated with fear—primal and stark.

On June 30, 2011, I sent an email with a far more optimistic tone than I was feeling.

> Apparently, life isn't just a bowl of kidneys or it
> would be easier to get one.
> I thought I'd bring you up to speed on what has
> been happening with me—mainly acquiring a kidney
> and learning patience.

Many of you know (and some of you don't) that a tumor was discovered on my sister's kidney and I had to come up with a plan B for a donor.

I've been so blessed. Three heroes have stepped forward for testing: my sister and my cousins John and Ken. Their generosity has been nothing short of a miracle to me. John was ruled out, and now after a myriad of tests and screenings, Ken has been ruled out at the final stage.

My sister is now being brought back as a candidate to donate. She's scheduled for an appointment on July 20. We hope a final determination will be made about her being a candidate shortly thereafter. The issue is that any possible risk of cancer must be ruled out in the kidney she would give me. If she's good to go, the surgery could be at the end of July. Here's a summary of what to expect based on the information I've been given:

The transplant itself will require four to six days in the hospital with a couple in ICU.

The overall recovery will be four to six weeks, which is typical for abdominal surgery, meaning no driving or lifting. Postsurgical symptoms and issues include but aren't limited to pain, nausea, acne, and a bigger head (seriously, from the steroids and— REALLY!—have you seen the size of my head?). They promise me they'll be able to deal with these symptoms and that they subside after a while. And by the way, along with the loss of my vanity, no more sun worshipping (I'll be sixty-five times more likely to get skin cancer because of the immune-suppressant medications) or sushi and undercooked meat (bacteria). Oh well . . . .

The initial few weeks after the surgery are crucial in order to avoid acute rejection of the kidney. From everything I've learned, the medicos have this process down, but it will require daily testing and frequent visits to the hospital for testing.

If things go well, I should be teaching my classes in the fall and dancing at Emily's wedding on October 1.

Thanks for your love, kindness, and support the past six months. Please keep sending it my way a little longer. It has made this journey bearable. I have been humbled many times by your goodness and care.

I'm looking forward to celebrating my new kidney with you in the coming months.

The responses were heartwarming and brought additional offers of a kidney.

Stewing in my own juices and feeling sorry for myself, an idea emerged from the chaos. What about Bret, the young man from Ohio who had offered me a kidney last March? I already knew we shared the same blood type. Ruminating about this option, I realized Bret might be the last egg in the basket for me. He was the last person I could contact before pulling the fire alarm. I was at the end of the rope, dangling and scared.

I decided to contact Bret through Emily and her soon-to-be husband, Terry. Audrey agreed. I needed to know if he was still serious about his offer. Terry called him, asking if he could come by for a beer and talk with him about giving me a kidney. Bret's response, which we soon learned was characteristic of his personality, was that Terry could come by for a beer, but he was already certain about donating a kidney. On his own and unprompted, Bret had already watched the transplant procedure on the internet.

When I heard that, I smiled. *Who is this guy?*

The cavalry was coming, and they all looked like Bret.

THE LAST MAN STANDING

*"Miracle" is simply the wonder of the unique that points us back
to the wonder of the everyday.*

—MAURICE FRIEDMAN

Bret Williams is certainly one of the more remarkable and intriguing
people I've ever encountered. Using iconic references from my own
generation, my initial impression was that he was the Marlboro Man,
Clint Eastwood, and John Wayne all rolled into one. More contemporary
references might include Chris Evans as Captain America or Charlie
Simms, Colonel Slade's babysitter with natural integrity in *Scent of a
Woman* (Chris O'Donnell played Simms, and Al Pacino was Slade).

Describing Bret as the strong, silent type was an understatement.
But I soon discovered he was sensitive, caring, and altruistic. Bret's
concealed strengths—a strong ethical code, kindness, and courage—
laid the foundation for him to even consider donating a kidney to me, let
alone actually do it. But an in-depth explanation of his decision wasn't
readily forthcoming. Bret was and is a man of action rather than words.

Back in March when Bret first offered his kidney, I wondered why
a twenty-seven-year-old single guy wanted to give me, a total stranger,
his kidney. Six months later, I still didn't know the answer. I might never

truly know or understand Bret's reasons for this amazing gift. I doubt most living donors can explain the reasons they donate. Why should Bret be any different? Later, I asked Bret about it because I wanted to include his perspective in his own words rather than mine. He told me his parents raised him to help others if he could. Consequently, because he had two kidneys, he could certainly give me one. His words and beliefs were simple, direct, powerful, and overwhelmingly beautiful.

Initially, I thought Bret was a friend of Emily and Terry. I believed they must know him well, or they must be at least casual friends with him. I eagerly searched for some connection to explain his generosity. I wanted there to be some order, some reason for offering me his kidney. I later discovered Bret was in Terry's broad social circle; he was "one of the guys" who went to a hunting camp near Chautauqua, New York, every Thanksgiving to hunt deer. A close friendship with Terry wasn't Bret's motivation; Terry barely knew him. I needed to, and learned to, accept and live with the ambiguity of how he came to give me a kidney.

Bret was actually a friend of Terry's dad. After retirement, Terry Sr. owned a neighborhood bar on the outskirts of Cleveland. He became friends with Bret when he would stop by for a beer after work. This initial contact eventually led to Bret, a jack-of-all-trades, doing odd jobs for Terry Sr. at the bar. From this connection, a friendship developed. In a casual conversation in March, Terry Sr. mentioned to Bret that his son's future bride's father needed a kidney (which is mouthful to say, let alone what it implied). As I understand it, Bret immediately offered to give me one of his kidneys. Confusing? Convoluted? Shocking? Strange? Miraculous? Wonderful? *Yes.* These reactions accurately describe my feelings about the original transaction that led to my acquiring a kidney. However peculiar the origin, the result was remarkable.

How miraculous that I was able to recuperate Bret's initial offer and avoid making the biggest mistake of my life. Equally momentous was that Bret never wavered, he never lost interest or wandered off. He never changed his mind. Bret's astonishing persistence, resolve, and dependability frame my entire story. More than likely, without his unbendable heart, my outcome would have been vastly different. I almost missed what I wanted the most. The reality of Bret remaining steadfastly resolute, even with my initial refusal of his offer, led me to wonder if other forces were at work. Perhaps my destiny awaited me all along.

In *Scent of a Woman*, Colonel Slade (who is blind) dances with a young and beautiful partner. After a breathtaking, scintillating tango, she tells him he dances amazingly. He responds, "I'm in the amazing business." Over the years, this line became part of our family lore. We use it to mark an incredibly kind or otherwise spectacular act. Bret and all donors are truly in the amazing business.

I wanted to understand the phenomenon of donating at a deeper level. Why do donors donate? I was hard-pressed to imagine a bolder, more life-giving act. To my knowledge, little is written on the subject of being a living donor. Only Suzanne F. Ruff's *The Reluctant Donor* comes to mind as a discussion of what it's like. In the form of research or subjective accounts, there's a scarcity of information that explores or explains why a person gives another person their organ. Individuals might have personal reasons, but knowledge of broader, shared reasons is absent. Donation as a living donor is an act without apparent explanation in human behavior. Yet it happens all the time, all over the country and all over the world. I recently heard a television news story by a Chicago station that described a grocery store cashier giving a kidney to a customer. The *New York Times* has reported that living-donor donations are happening more frequently as technology helps streamline multiple transplants in which a donor volunteers a kidney on behalf of a recipient for whom he or she isn't a match, but then donates to someone else in need, thus setting off a chain of transplants. These are called *kidney chains* or *kidney swaps*.

I wondered then—and still do—if Bret and others like him have a gene for unselfishness. The other individuals who offered me a kidney also did so with little hesitation, responding positively and affirmatively. From these incredible offers, I developed a mental template with four tiers of would-be donors: 1) Those, like Bret, Roseann, and Ken, whose offer was immediate and automatic; 2) those who offered more slowly with some hesitation; 3) those who were reluctant or measured but would step up if there were no other alternatives; and 4) those who would but were not able to donate by some type of limiting factor, like age or health or fear. Obviously, my categorizations aren't research based. They're suppositions that emerged from my attempt to understand the profound generosity of a person giving someone else an organ.

Bret randomly emerging when I was in dire need was puzzling to say the least. It felt like a miracle. I considered if my getting his kidney was merely random or ultimately chance. Was it really just luck? Perhaps. It would be easy to write it off as mere coincidence, but it felt like more than that. Then and now.

Although I talk about Bret in the context of "finding a donor," in a way, Bret found me. Our connection was made by people I'd only begun to know. From a different point of view, my situation presented Bret with an opportunity to do what he was meant to do, become a hero for me. I came to believe Bret was going to do something life-giving for someone at some point in his life. (A post-transplant email from Bret's sister later confirmed this idea.) Bret was on a trajectory to help someone in need. He was meant to be someone's champion. Our paths intersected. I became the beneficiary of his incredible goodness and altruism. At some level, the momentums of our lives brought us together, and I got extremely lucky. My life and the quality of it would be profoundly changed as a result of this inspiring connection.

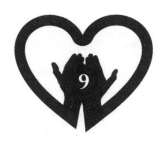

DANCING WITH DOCTORS, HOSPITALS, AND MYSELF

Kindness, I've discovered, is everything in life.

—Isaac Bashevis Singer

After Bret gave the green light, things shifted at the Transplant Clinic. I had another donor lined up and ready to go. Bret immediately called Kathy Davis, answered questions about his health and medical history, and passed the screening. Vials were then sent to him so that he could send his blood back to be tested for tissue matches and antibodies. The process of receiving the vials, getting the blood test, and returning them took about two weeks—and then there was a ten-day waiting period to determine if any antigens emerged.

I wondered if the medical staff had ever experienced a patient family like us. We acted like we were the ones in charge, thinking we were being "good" consumers and self-advocates. Luckily, those who were truly in charge granted us this courtesy, perhaps thinking we were being a collective pain in the ass. Whatever the case, the staff acted professionally and patiently.

With Bret rapidly progressing through testing and looking like an excellent donor, our thinking shifted to Emily's wedding. We wanted to have the transplant at the end of August so I could walk Emily down the aisle on October 1 unencumbered and Bret's life could reset to normal as soon as possible. Dr. Becker was sympathetic but cautioned us about traveling so soon after a major surgical event. When Bret was approved, I wrote to Dr. Becker:

> Minutes ago, I received some wonderful news that Bret Williams's blood tests cleared and he was approved as a possible donor for me. Hallelujah! What great news.
>
> Unfortunately, he was told by Kathy Davis that he can't be scheduled to get the additional medical tests until August 31. Ugh. Double ugh! I had hoped that the transplant would be done on August 30, if not sooner. Can this be true? A three-week wait? Why so long?
>
> I just got off the phone with Bret and he's ready to go. I'm ready. Is there any way he can be tested next week? In our last email communication you indicated that the scheduling problems were often the result of complications with the donor. This is obviously not the case in my situation. Bret would be there tomorrow if you approved it.
>
> I want to ask you to be my advocate in this situation and intervene to see if the tests can be scheduled earlier.
>
> I know you have my best interest at heart so please do what you can on my behalf. Now is the time for all good (great) surgeons to come to the aid of their patients. Please don't let scheduling be the reason I wait until October.
>
> Thank you and thank you more if you can bend the river and change the culture in your department.

Dr. Becker replied a few hours later:

> We have been making several calls to try to
> facilitate your potential donor's work-up. Your
> insurance requires that many of the potential
> donor's studies be completed in Chicago rather
> than sending from another center. Therefore,
> it takes a lot of coordinating to minimize the
> inconvenience to your friend and multiple visits.
> I'm sure you want to advocate for the best for your
> donor and I'm sure you understand that this is all
> medical risk to that individual.

The next morning Dr. Becker added: "Please keep in mind that I am still hesitant to promise that you will be free to travel in early October at this point. It is very quick to have such strenuous activity as a wedding."

Although I chose to ignore it at the time, Becker's comment foreshadowed what came into play very soon. But the entire medical staff came through for us in this regard. We moved toward a late August date for surgery. In that moment, I was thrilled to say the least.

Waiting—and waiting some more—is, from the patient's point of view, the primary characteristic of health care, medicine, and hospitals. Searching for a donor and eventually getting a transplant increased the waiting time exponentially. Time slowed to a crawl as each donor emerged and then receded, and another emerged and then receded. I considered myself a relatively patient person, but in this situation my tolerance was challenged continuously. The underlying battle with patience was really about control. Finding a balance between control and acceptance was a fight, even a war, which was constantly raging inside me. Ultimately, I realized I had no control over Bret becoming a donor or the results of his medical tests; but with my life itself at stake, I tried to influence the outcome to whatever extent possible.

After getting the news that our blood was compatible and that we could move to the next step, the lost momentum that accompanied Ken's and my sister's rejection was restored. Hope and optimism returned. As happy as my family, friends, and I were, we knew from previous experience not to get carried away. I wanted to celebrate the good news, but stay in the moment, minimizing any attachment to the outcome. I recognized that things could go either way at this point. *Stay grounded*, I told myself over and over.

With Bret's smooth progression through the myriad of initial tests and interviews and my increasing comfort with his being ultimately being cleared, a considerable amount of introspection emerged on my part about who I was as a person. My coping abilities were tested, and the strain of the search was increasingly transparent. Even though Audrey and I were committed to a proactive approach, we also knew finding a donor was typically a three- to five-year process. We were clearly bucking the odds. While staunchly maintaining our belief that I would find a kidney, we did our best to cultivate a sense of balance, not wanting our moods to swing too high or too low.

Bret and his kidney were the best option for my health and survival: a twenty-seven-year-old kidney was better than a fifty-five-year-old kidney (as in the case of Roseann) or a fifty-year-old kidney (in the case of Ken). Realism and practicality were integral parts of our perspective. And now the doors of hope and optimism were pushed wide open with the confirmation of our blood compatibility.

The next series of medical tests for Bret was less daunting. In fact, he was an extraordinary physical specimen: young, incredibly healthy, and, as it turned out, with "perfect" kidneys. One of the post-transplant nephrologists, Dr. James Chon, later described the kidney Bret gave me as "pristine." The next stage was bringing Bret to Chicago for the array of more in-depth medical tests that would ultimately determine his viability as a donor.

Our first conversation consisted of me asking Bret if he was sure he wanted to donate a kidney and then profusely thanking him when he assured me he was. During the conversation, some of his qualities became evident: his kindness, his compassion for someone in need, his moral clarity, and his fearlessness. On the surface Bret was a macho guy, a man's man. What I quickly discovered was his goodness—not only in word but also in action. Bret spoke directly. When I asked why he was doing this, he replied, "You needed a kidney. I have two. So why wouldn't I give you one?" Once he made a decision, he adamantly stuck to it. He evidently had a strong will to do what he perceived to be the "right" thing. Bret never wavered. He took a moral stance then delivered on it by being my donor.

In a guestbook entry on my CaringBridge site (an online platform for sharing individuals' health-related stories) after the transplant surgery, Bret's sister said she always thought Bret would give someone an arm or leg. As it turned out, Bret gave a kidney. Her statement helped ease my doubts. Early on, I worried Bret acted on a whim or made the decision arbitrarily. Over time I realized his resolution was an integral part of who he was, and giving me a kidney wasn't an impulsive decision he might later regret.

Our second phone conversation, just like the first, started with me asking him if he was sure he wanted to give me a kidney. His affirmative reply was even more emphatic. With my doubt quieted, the conversation moved to working out a date for him to fly to Chicago. I told him to buy the ticket, and I'd reimburse him. And I said I'd pick him up at the airport and take him to the hospital. The next day Emily called. Bret had contacted her to tell her he didn't have a credit card to pay for the ticket. Emily, gracefully and without hesitation, bought the ticket.

Emily's action avoided a potential problem and further engaged her in the process. At Terry's suggestion, Emily accompanied Bret to Chicago and stood by him throughout the entire testing process. I always knew Emily was special, but for her to step up, unsolicited, and help get Bret to Chicago was an exquisite example of unconditional love. I was the beneficiary of tremendous compassion from numerous people. The transcendent quality of what was developing persisted, and somehow many independent variables were interacting positively on my behalf. Forces converged that guided our efforts toward success. Numerous people contributed to help me get a kidney. I laughed at my efforts to control things and marveled at how I was essentially being carried by peoples' love and compassion. My journey, which began with fear and trepidation, was developing into a marvelous story, filled with grace and beauty.

Later in a CaringBridge entry, I wrote that everyone should have an opportunity to experience the unconditional love I felt during this time. I believe there is a fundamental human need to be loved unconditionally from at least one other person in our lives (an idea I first heard expressed by Elisabeth Kübler-Ross when I had brought her to Oakton for a lecture). Experiencing unconditional love in the way I did throughout my experience—I might not have believed it if I hadn't lived it.

Bret moved briskly through the testing that week. The doctors and nurses were impressed by his extraordinary physical condition. As each day passed, my prospects of getting a kidney rapidly escalated. My hopes went through the roof. Audrey and I were giddy.

One curious aspect of Bret's early hospital experience was a barrage of questions from almost every medical person he encountered—was he being coerced, bribed, or paid to give me his kidney? He finally told one of the medical staff members to stop it, that he was insulted by this constant interrogation. I understood the dilemma. Donors needed to be protected. Why would a twenty-seven-year-old stranger perform such a noble act? My situation was unusual in that my family and I were very involved with Bret from the start. Most donors are kept at a distance and have anonymity. At one point after being inundated with questions, Bret wouldn't even let Emily buy him lunch. The process wasn't easy on Bret, even with a supportive, compassionate medical staff.

After the first day, we decided to celebrate by taking Bret to the local Evanston steakhouse. Enjoying a wonderful meal, we were festive and happy. Bret started to relax and assimilate into the family. It was easy to see that he was a good guy and down to earth—a bit rough and tumble on the surface, but kind and gentle underneath. It helped to laugh with him, letting the awkwardness of the hospital and the overall heaviness of the situation dissipate.

Bret passed the medical tests with flying colors. I had a donor. His success was noteworthy, given our recent donor history. Meanwhile my creatinine continued to increase. Although Dr. Nash thought there was no imminent danger, it was a reminder that the clock was ticking.

Bret and I still wanted the transplant surgery done immediately. Even though Dr. Becker discouraged doing it before Emily's impending wedding, I decided to push to get the surgery done at the end of August. Despite the doctors at Audrey's workplace agreeing with Becker to wait, I was determined to support Bret's preference to get it over with.

Audrey wasn't happy with my decision. For the first time in the process we were out of sync. She was worried and anxious about the wedding. Even though Emily and Terry were extremely supportive of whatever I chose to do, Audrey felt differently. She was focused on the best medical choice. I argued that Bret wanted to get the surgery over, and I did not want to wait two more months to have this part of my life in the rearview mirror. I believed waiting longer might do me in completely. Audrey relented, but her stress was undeniable.

After contacting Kathy Davis to reschedule the surgery—and then asking Dr. Becker to intervene on my behalf, which she did—the plan for surgery at the end of August was put into motion. But even with Becker's consent for the earlier date, I remained anxious and confused.

The strain between Audrey and I was increasing. Fortunately, I came to my senses and got a grip. As this process of determining a surgery date was unfolding, a chance meeting at a wedding (of Haley Wadsworth, one of Emily's friends) with one of the emergency room doctors from the University of Chicago, Dr. David Howze, led me to rethink my situation and reverse my direction. In my eagerness to get things over with, I had denied my own anxiety about the surgery. I simply wasn't ready. I needed more time to emotionally prepare myself. I also reconsidered my insensitivity to Audrey's feelings. When this reality hit, I had to undo what I'd done only days earlier. On August 19, I meekly emailed Dr. Becker:

> With the way this process is developing, my discussion with other transplant patients, Dr. Howze's opinion, and at the risk of Kathy Davis wanting to strangle me, I've come to the conclusion that your initial recommendation of waiting until after October 1 (after my daughter's wedding) may be the most prudent and best way to proceed. As much as the waiting has been stressful, the added drama of potentially not being able to travel at the end of September has led me to conclude that, given that my current health status is stable, the best decision is to wait until after October 1 to have the transplant surgery.
>
> I apologize to you and all concerned for having pushed the system to get Bret tested early and certainly acknowledge everyone's efforts as above and beyond in accomplishing that.
>
> So assuming you agree and can accommodate my choice, I'll stay the course until I hear from you officially next week and make all the necessary preparations for a Tuesday in October, perhaps October 11?

Dr. Becker graciously replied: "I think this is a wise decision. Please enjoy your daughter's wedding and we will plan for a date to follow, hoping all is approved at our meeting."

Feeling foolish and humble after finally resolving the surgical date issue, I was relieved. Letting go of control led to a happy outcome. When I got out of my own way, good things happened. Although I was a slow learner, I finally got it.

I ate, deservedly so, a large slice of humble pie. There were no recriminations from the medical staff. No one said *I told you so*. Audrey was tremendously relieved and appreciative. Emily was relieved, although she never said that, always echoing her constant refrain, "Whatever is best for you, Dad." As it turned out, my change of mind and heart was singularly the best decision I made about my surgical process. Judging by my actual recovery, I could never have traveled or been able to participate in my daughter's wedding at the level I did. Delaying the surgery date paid countless dividends.

The only negative was Bret's disappointment. He graciously agreed, but I knew he didn't want to wait. Even though his immediate responses were "Do whatever is best for you" and "I understand," I discovered much later that the change in date created problems for him. It was difficult for Bret to disappoint me or my family.

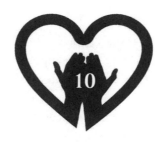

STAYING THE COURSE

The aim of life is to live, and to live means to be aware, joyously,
drunkenly, serenely, divinely aware.

—HENRY MILLER

Even though the wedding would bring us joy and my guilt-filled revision of the surgery date was complete, there were still two more months of waiting to be dealt with. It seemed like an eternity. Other issues remained and persisted. Even though I chose to do so, waiting was going to be a struggle. With that much time left to go, immersing myself in the most normal life available seemed like an excellent idea. What surprised me were the benefits I received during this time.

On August 24, I sent an email with the subject line "Donor Approved."

Dear family and friends,

The long summer of waiting appears to be over.
It's with a joyful heart that I'm contacting you
to let you know that, as of Monday evening, I have
an officially approved donor. The stress of waiting
and not knowing, and the ups and downs of being so
close seem to have passed. Onward to the challenge
of transplant surgery and then recovery.

Bret Williams—a friend of my daughter Emily and her husband-to-be's father and now my best friend—has amazingly stepped up, passed all the screenings and tests and consented to give me one of his kidneys. Wow! This new reality is still overwhelming for me and my family. At Bret's last appointment with a nephrologist at UChicago on Friday he was told he is a "better-than-textbook match." I'm not sure what this means medically, but I love the sound of it.

Because of Emily's impending nuptials and at the recommendation of my surgeon, I've decided to wait to have the transplant surgery until after October 1, most likely October 11. I'll keep you posted when the exact date is determined.

I want to again honor the wonderful people who offered to donate earlier: my friends Randy and Susan; a stranger in a restaurant; my brother-in-law, Al; my nephew, Michael; my cousins John and Ken; and my sister, Roseann (twice). I can't help but feel that without them and the unfolding of this series of events, I wouldn't be in the place I am now—about to get a living-donor kidney. I'll always have a special place in my heart for their generosity, kindness, and compassion. They're incredibly special and unique people.

So after a year devoted to finding a kidney, I get to have surgery. There's a bit of irony in this—struggle, hope, and rejection lead to fear and surgery. How fortunate can a guy be? Really. It wasn't that long ago that the outcome for this wasn't very good and certainly not all that appealing. I'm blessed to have this opportunity. My awesome surgeon at the UChicago, Dr. Yolanda Becker, keeps talking to me about having a twenty-seven-year-old kidney. I hope she's right.

> Thank you for all your kindness and support
> these past months. I'm looking forward to facing the
> challenge of surgery and coming back stronger and
> better with a renewed body and attitude.

> With love and gratitude, Greg

As it turned out, the upsides of postponing were abundant. Ironically, but typical of my adventure, when I surrendered control, allowing myself to go with the flow, positive things happened. Being open and fluid allowed me to absorb the plentiful support available. Even though my mental and physical energy were fading due to end-stage renal disease, the prevailing reality of my current situation was that I never really *felt* sick in the way one would with the flu or a comparable illness. I did, however, feel extremely fatigued. Every day after work, I would immediately nap. Despite my depleted state, I attempted to live a relatively normal life, including work, socializing, exercising at a limited capacity, and, of course, preparing for the wedding. My reduced routine provided the necessary space to ready myself emotionally for what was ahead. Each day, little by little, I prepared myself for the scalpel and confronted the fears of what might go wrong—and the energy-giving possibilities of what could go right.

I found solace in working and teaching, despite my worries that I'd find it a terrible ordeal. Commitment to a daily routine that included outside responsibilities and having a place to go distracted me and yielded yet another marvelous gift. Curiously, functioning in settings where I wasn't watching my own navel and stewing in my own preoperative juices was the best medicine.

In person and via emails, the outpouring of support at work was wonderful. Without a doubt, my colleagues' compassion made a tremendous difference in my state of mind and being. I understood in a new way Lou Gehrig's speech at the end of his career in Yankee Stadium—the one that begins, "Today, I consider myself the luckiest man on the face of this earth." I didn't foresee or expect the compassionate concern coming from my colleagues. The challenge was to stay open to it and be nurtured by it.

A beautiful example of this came from Peg Lee, Oakton Community College's president, and Joi Smith, the vice president of student affairs. Although I had accrued enough sick days that my surgery and recovery wouldn't be a work issue, Peg and Joi reiterated, "Do what you need to do to take care of yourself." Their support eradicated any lingering work-related anxiety. Even now, reflecting on their kindness touches my heart.

Unfortunately, Audrey had the opposite experience at her job. This reversal of circumstances and conditions each of us experienced contained more than a touch of irony. She worked in a hospital—a place you would think would show more compassion about the time required for healing and recovery for both the patient and family. But the bureaucratic nature of the hospital and the rigid structure of her department—which demonstrated its values by awarding bonuses based on attendance rather than quality of work—were creating an often unbearable strain for her at this time. Besides dealing with my situation, Audrey was continuously coping with a system that was usually more rigid than flexible, with the occasional exception of empathethc and kind acts by some of the doctors and fellow CRNAs. While waiting for surgery, I did not know or realize that in many ways my ordeal was more difficult for her than me. Over time, the toll extracted caused her to get seriously ill the following winter and spring. Caregivers often pay a high price when they continuously make someone else their priority. Audrey was no different.

I had lunch every Monday with my closest-knit group of friends, a.k.a. the Knuckleheads: Cary Schawel, Paul Johnson, and Joe Kotowski (and Jan Thompson-Wilda when she was around). Laughter dominated our weekly encounter. Our routine kept me grounded, sane, and distracted. The ongoing banter and teasing never let me sink too low or take myself too seriously. We had a running gag going about Joe being a blood-type match with me, which made him a possible donor. But because he was so anxious about seeing his own blood, he couldn't tolerate thinking about donating a kidney. At any moment, one of us might ask him if he was going to give me a kidney.

I told Joe, all kidding aside, that I had no problems or qualms about his not being a donor. When I asked someone for a kidney, I genuinely didn't have any investment in the outcome individual by individual, I didn't personalize my expectations of the person, and I tried to silence any remorse expressed. Getting a kidney required that it be freely given or not at all. Although people in my situation needed to ask, each person has the inherent right of saying no for any reason. My life or health is no more important than another's life or health. I had absolute clarity about that.

It is important to note that I believed any number of my friends would not let me die or ultimately go without a kidney if things degenerated. In all of our joking and teasing, I believed others had my back. I took comfort knowing I was protected. Friends—during a time fraught with fear, anxiety, and risk—were essential. This simple truth was another gift to me.

During the time I was awaiting the transplant, I was also planning my retirement for the summer of 2012. After thirty-one years, I would "head for the barn" for good. The emergence of my disease validated my decision, made three years earlier, to retire. This health crisis removed any doubt I had about ending my career at the relatively young age of fifty-nine. Choosing to retire was a good decision. I mused that I could live with calling it quits on the career front—literally and figuratively.

The pressure of wanting to put closure to my professional life intensified the impending reality of transplant surgery. I didn't want to end my career on a stretcher: weak, broken, or disabled. For close to forty years, I derived a life-giving energy from teaching. To have it taken from me because of my kidney disease or inability to recover fast enough would have been a crippling defeat. Let's face it, fear can motivate; it certainly did in my case. It became extremely important to me to finish with a flourish. My goal: function as best I could before the surgery and then return in January for a final semester. Having a clear professional goal sharpened my resolve going into the surgery and fueled my recovery.

The strain of dealing with two major life stressors—a medical crisis and retirement—necessitated an attitude adjustment. I needed help and support. What inspired and allowed me to cope with my complex situation was a concoction of various factors—friendship, laughter, love, support—that came into play on a regular basis, changing frequently, day to day or hour to hour. As my personal strengths and incentives waned and I weakened, I allowed myself to be carried by those around me. Most of my motivation came from Audrey, a family member, or a close friend. But many contributed to my overall well-being at different times and in different ways. Sometimes a simple smile of inquiry about how things were going fueled my efforts. Having a support system provided numerous reasons to carry on and continually strengthened and renewed my determination.

Rescheduling the surgery continued to pay dividends. I came to cherish the extra time. My work was meaningful, and it distracted me from my date with destiny. Anxiety crept into my mind, but not while I was working. The extra weeks allowed me to focus on emotionally preparing for the actual surgery, which helped me maintain a calmer, more peaceful state of mind. A sense of clarity emerged during those last weeks and carried me to the actual procedure.

The impending wedding was also a counterpoint to the stress. Emily's enthusiasm and happiness was contagious. The joy in her daily call describing the charming details of wedding planning was a welcome interruption; the calls got me out of myself and gave Audrey some much-needed relief from the burden she was carrying—me. Emily's excitement was life-affirming. Realizing that life does go on, and there's more to it than fighting disease, sustained me. Life is an irrepressible force undiminished by individual struggle and worry. Soon many hearts would be filled with the elation, regeneration, and love that a wedding brings. Our collective focus on that event meant I wasn't the center of the universe all the time, and being out of the spotlight was a welcome escape. Self-absorption is a crippling curse, and I was no exception. The wedding commotion and being the father of the bride kept many demons at bay.

Emily's wedding on October 1, 2011, in Chautauqua, New York, was filled with joy and love. Almost two hundred family members and friends joined us to make the four-day weekend one to remember. Thankfully, I held up surprisingly well. Although my energy was questionable at times, I only had one really bad stretch—after the rehearsal dinner. I went to bed early feeling weak and apprehensive about surviving the big day. Luckily, I woke up excited and ready to go. Even though it was cool and rainy and the temperature was falling, the wedding went off without a hitch. The ceremony was glorious. The bride and groom washed all those in attendance with love and warmth. I couldn't have been happier or prouder that day.

When I gave the father-of-the-bride speech at the reception, I shared something Emily told us two months earlier when getting a kidney was still unresolved. With typical grace, Emily said, "The weather could be bad as long as Dad got a kidney and got healthy again." Her prophetic words about the weather came true. As fog enveloped the tent and the rain-saturated grass squished beneath my feet, I reminded Emily of what she'd said. "The cool, damp, and rainy weather was good for me but not so good for you on your wedding day," I announced to all present. Tears flowed freely. Looking back, it is hard to decide who got the better deal: me, Emily, or Terry.

I was swept away by the intensity of the moment. Weddings do that sort of thing, right? The shared energy felt transcendent. I've never had an out-of-body experience before, and this was as close to one as I will probably ever get. I felt as if I were part of something bigger than my own travails. Paradoxically, I felt small and big—humbled and expanded—at the same time. I felt a true sense of wonder.

After the wedding, I continued to feel I was participating in something larger and greater than my own troubles. I had a strong sense of egolessness. It wasn't as dramatic or intense as at the wedding, but it was overt enough that I recognized it and was affected by it. I saw my life and my struggle differently after the wedding. When the stakes are life and death, the insights are intense. Seeing and experiencing life from this perspective was unexpected and another precious gift.

THE COUNTDOWN

Life is not a problem to solved, but a reality to be experienced.

—Søren Kierkegaard

With the wedding over, I was ten days away from my transplant surgery. We were in the homestretch. This event dominating my life, this event that was both sought and feared—was close at hand. The idea of the impending surgery was at once paralyzing and invigorating; my head was spinning with dozens of simultaneous thoughts and feelings.

On the physical plane, I was exhausted. Sleeping, even naps, did little or no good. I woke tired. The one certainty was that I had to put one foot in front of the other and keep moving forward—literally. On a more spiritual level, I was acutely aware of the relentlessness of time. The Latin phrase *tempus fugit* (time flies) took on a new meaning. The future, whether desired or feared, always arrived. I just needed to persevere. I kept repeating different mantras to myself: *Don't give up. Don't quit. Don't fail.* My goal was to show up at the UChicago hospital on Wednesday, October 12, at 7:00 a.m. Everything after that was out of my control. I looked forward to that surrender.

If only it were that simple. I complicated the situation with thoughts and questions about dying. Previously when I considered that possibility, I ruminated about it without resolution by ignoring, minimizing, or adopting a meditative response—and certainly not lingering for more than a few fleeting moments. Now, with the clock ticking, I was forced to confront in a new and vulnerable way the possibility of my own demise or impairment.

Struggling with the possibility of dying was contradicted by my confidence that I would survive surgery. Dr. Becker reassured me they had "perfected this procedure." This kind of certainty from a doctor of her stature was rare, and I was convinced. I trusted Becker and the team—and especially Audrey, who voiced similar confidence—implicitly and without reservation. Despite the reassurances, my perseverating thoughts continued. When confusion prevailed, Audrey reassured me.

A week before the surgery, I pressed Audrey with my concerns. Does everyone facing a serious surgery have these fears and doubts? Her years of experience offered helpful perspectives: *These fears are real for the person enduring them. The surgery has great risk and uncertainty. There is value in confronting my fears.* Sharing my worries created intimacy and relieved the "craziness" that can result from internalizing thoughts and fears. Processing the fear restored some semblance of balance, and it helped turn my vulnerability into strength.

My primary concern was if I should say good-bye to the people most important to me—my wife and children. I envisioned myself having an emotional interaction with Audrey and each of my children—Sarah, Emily, and Luke—at my hospital bedside. I would tell each of them how much I love them and ask them to forgive my mistakes. I thought I might need to make peace with them. Or perhaps I'd seen too many movies? Regardless, I wanted to thank them for being in my life and for the gifts they'd given me. Mostly I wanted to tell them how much I loved them. A crisis-fueled circumstance isn't a requirement for saying "I love you," but it does add urgency.

Because of Becker's and Audrey's reassurances, I chose not to consider the possibility of surgical death and the resulting emotional good-byes. Nonetheless, I was genuinely confronting my mortality. Making sense of my life and facing my possible end was paramount and essential, even if it was done only internally. This crisis of meaning was life-affirming. Not only was I navigating the surgical drama, I was about to have a landmark birthday, sixty, just two weeks later. I found myself newly aware of how fragile and short life is. Granted, I'm not the first to ruminate on those truths, but when life's parameters are so vivid and real, it's impossible to trivialize or distance them through philosophizing. An incredible opportunity was presenting itself— rather than defeat and death, I had a chance at *life* and *renewal*. I started to ask myself: *What should I do with this new life I'm being given?*

My preoperative appointment with Becker happened a week before the surgery. One test—an ultrasound to determine the placement of the new kidney and to check the size of my old ones— remained. The resident in the ultrasound room did a double take when she saw me, and then quickly excused herself. When she returned, she said, "You looked so good I thought you might be the donor instead of the recipient." We laughed. I had that going for me—I still looked "marvelous" despite end-stage renal disease. My old, diseased kidneys were approximately two (right one) and three (left one) times larger than normal. For a person my size, a normal kidney is about the size of my fist. My old kidneys were significantly larger and hardly functioning at all, at less than 10 percent. My creatinine was 7.6 (it would rise to more than 8.0 the day of the surgery). The need for dialysis loomed large; fortunately, my surgery date was near.

Dr. Becker was her usual charming and brilliant self, and she spent a long time with us that day. I felt completely confident in her abilities. She eliminated the possibility of taking out one or both of my old kidneys, even though I had initially requested the double nephrectomy at my first clinic visit. She convinced us that the risks for excessive bleeding and infection from the removal of my old kidneys were too high. I was getting a "perfect" kidney from a young, healthy donor, which precipitously increased the odds for a successful transplant. But excessive bleeding or clotting during the surgery while attempting to remove my old kidneys would force the immediate termination of the transplant. Why jeopardize the procedure? Why complicate my wonderful chance of success? We left the appointment in wholehearted agreement with her.

During this same meeting and consultation, Becker also revealed something nonmedical that further enhanced her status in my eyes. Typically, transplant surgeries at the UChicago hospital are on Tuesdays. I wondered why my surgery was scheduled for Wednesday. When asked, her response brought a smile to my face—it was her son's eleventh birthday, and she was spending Tuesday with him. Not wanting to hold two priorities in her head, she assured me that with his day complete, she would be totally present for me and surgery. I loved her honesty and her love for her son. In that simple moment, Dr. Yolanda Becker became real.

With a week to "Transplant Day," I cozied up to my established routine. Thank God for habit. With the last few details in order, a calm settled in for both Audrey and me. The final lap was soon to be run. I could almost see the finish line.

HAPPY TRANSPLANT
SURGERY EVE

I worked the Monday and Tuesday before my surgery. What else was I
going to do? Audrey decided to work in order to save her days off for
later. I taught and said farewell to friends and students. I soaked up
every drop of support available from anyone and everyone who offered
it. My last gallows-humor lunch with the Knuckleheads was filled with
laugher. I left Oakton that last day feeling optimistic. My impending
surgery felt more like I was waiting to fly somewhere rather than I was
about to fall off a cliff.

Emily arrived a few days earlier, Sarah was on her way, and
Luke had returned from school and was already at home. Bret was
scheduled to come in Tuesday night. His arrival was simple . . . and
complicated. How fitting. He came carrying only an athletic bag with
a few clothes in it. He looked healthy and confident. Like General

Douglas MacArthur and the Terminator before him, he had returned. Thanks to my persistent and pesky insecurities, I wasn't entirely sure he would. My doubts weren't caused by anything Bret said or did. My continual questioning about whether the transplant was actually going to happen only stopped when I awoke with his kidney. Still, the gravity of the situation and my better nature led me to tell him the morning of the surgery that he could back out at any time. I told him there would be no hard feelings and that I would understand. Even as I swam in a pool of my own doubts, I wanted Bret to be as certain about his decision as humanly possible.

Losing control of my life and future had left me percolating with helplessness for months. I didn't know then how my feelings of vulnerability would stay with me in the coming months and even substantially increase. In the last few days and hours before surgery I felt like I was riding a wave that might suddenly break, heaving me into deep, dark water and leaving me to drown.

Bret's parents were planning to be at the hospital on Wednesday for his surgery. Initially, Bret intended to fly solo for it. We thought this was strange, but it was Bret's call. Nonetheless, we were relieved to know he'd agreed to have his family present. As we got to know him better, we realized Bret could neither be forced to do something nor pressured into changing once he'd made a decision. We could only trust and accept his choices about what he would and would not do. We also realized a part of Bret would always be mysterious.

The night before the surgery, the family assembled—Audrey, Sarah, Emily, Terry, Luke, Bret, and me. By now we considered Bret a part of our family. Emily and Sarah had accompanied Bret to the hospital earlier that day for his pre-op visit. All systems were go. We spent Tuesday evening talking and kidding around. Luke, although quiet and perhaps a bit overwhelmed, participated in the levity. His presence was essential and added to the overall mood, which was surprisingly relaxed. An unexpected ease emerged and replaced our collective anxiety. It was transparent that we were all pulling in the same direction.

Just before retiring for the night, Sarah brilliantly decided to open an account on CaringBridge, a blog that allows families to post the progress of a patient during their medical intervention, so family members and friends can share news about the ailing person. Sarah's decision evolved into one of the most incredible aspects of our common adventure. It provided an amazing support system for us during and after the transplant. People followed my progress through the malaise of hospitals, surgery, and recovery. Daily entries and responses became an integral part of our routine, bringing great joy to us as people responded with support, care, and love.

Here's the first entry, "The Night Before," posted on October 11, 2011, at 9:43 p.m.:

> Greetings from Evanston!
>
> The fam is sitting in the Native American Museum [the kids' nickname for my collection of native art] musing about the "big" day tomorrow and listening to the *Pulp Fiction* soundtrack. Some of us, not Bret or I, are having a glass of wine.
>
> It's almost like any other family gathering.
>
> We're about as ready as can be. Only about nine hours to kidney time.
>
> Thank you, thank you, thank you for all your wonderful responses to my emails. They're quite inspiring and heartwarming.
>
> All of you make such a difference in my life.
>
> Much gratitude, Sarah

Seemingly insignificant and only a nice thing to do at first, CaringBridge became a cornerstone of my adventure for the following year.

We had a pretty good and satisfying idea of what would transpire the following day. Bret would go to the hospital about an hour before me to be prepped for his surgery, which would start an hour before mine. As a final preparation, Bret and I washed ourselves before we went to bed and again in the morning with a powerful antiseptic. The removal of germs and bacteria seemed like an appropriate physical and psychological gesture. This emotional, symbolic purging of the old and defective would allow for a transformation to the new and healthy. As the evening came to its end, a somberness and quietness engulfed the house while we dispersed to make our attempts to sleep.

I was as ready as I could be. *Bring it on,* I thought. Lying in bed with Audrey beside me and with a heightened awareness of my skin, now sticky with residual antiseptic wash, I was comforted by the belief I was going to make it. *Show up. Stumble through. Survive.*

ANSWERING THE BELL

Do the thing we fear, and the death of fear is certain.

—RALPH WALDO EMERSON

Morning never arrived so quickly.

I slept surprisingly well the night before the transplant, but not very long. I was content to get any rest at all. The previous evening with my family created a kind of security and tranquility I'd never before experienced. Together, in the face of this extraordinary situation, they cast a serene light that overcame the darkness of my colossal anxiety.

As morning came, my nerves and fear emerged again. Despite my feeble attempt to hide it, my emotional condition was transparent. We prepared quickly and efficiently. Our ballet reminded me of the 1987 movie *Roxanne,* in which Steve Martin plays the fire chief of a volunteer fire department in a small Oregon town. The volunteer fire crew muddles through drills and rehearsals in a painful fashion, but when a real fire breaks out, they adroitly perform a choreographed dance as they ready themselves for a crisis. That morning, we were the firefighters responding to a five-alarm fire.

Driving down Chicago's Lake Shore Drive to the hospital was unexpectedly painless. Even the section through Grant Park in downtown Chicago, typically slow and even scary, was effortless. We were on a mission and nothing would deter us.

Arriving at the hospital, I was quiet, which is unusual for me. Generally, I'm outgoing and talkative with an active sense of humor. Not this day. Every so often the kids asked me if I was all right. They understood my silence gave away my preoccupation. I mumbled terse responses that I was fine or as good as could be expected. In fact, I was terrified, but I didn't want to make the experience harder for them by decompensating. But inside my head and body, I was a mess. My anxiety was palpable. My steps and speech were slowed, thinking I might collapse with any random step. Someone was always at my side to catch me if I stumbled.

Because I was preregistered, after a very brief check-in, I was off to get a CAT scan and then prepped for the first procedure. I needed to be led to Radiology because a personal fog was thickening around me. Navigating the hospital halls was like walking in a dream. I was cognizant of what was happening, but it was also like having an out-of-body experience. I observed myself going through this process. It felt otherworldly, even surreal. People and sounds were exaggerated. It seemed like I was floating from stop to stop rather than walking. The procedures went smoothly and the waiting was relatively short. The first glitch happened when I attempted to move my bowels. No luck. Little did I know then that this blunder would be a major problem after surgery.

The next stop was Interventional Radiology to have a central line inserted in my right upper chest. I didn't realize it at the time, but it was an unnecessary procedure. Someone assumed I was participating in a research study I'd declined two months earlier. Initially, Audrey thought it was merely a very conservative approach to a potential emergency that might occur during or after the surgery. I cooperated, but in retrospect I consider it one of the few errors made during my entire hospital stay. I was sedated for it, and the anesthesia was a welcome relief from my anxiety. During the procedure, Audrey shared the day's first CaringBridge entry:

> Well, I really don't like being on this side of things. Greg just went into Interventional Radiology to get a central line put in. Versed and fentanyl are his new best friends now; he had a smile on his face. We're told his surgery will start between 11:00 and 11:30. Hospital time is measured in dog years. The nurse anesthetist for the surgery, David Clanton (who used to work at Evanston), just came by—very reassuring. We brought smiley-face cookies for the surgical team, E-Town [Evanston] style. Keep the good vibes coming.
>
> Audrey

After the central-line procedure I felt woozy and dopey. But my silence and withdrawal were reversed. I turned quite talkative and silly while we waited for the main event.

There I was—in a curtained side room of Interventional Radiology waiting for the previous surgery to finish and for Becker to visit. My entire immediate family surrounded me. Lying there waiting, calmed by the sedation, my perception shifted. For the first time, I became aware of their nervousness and anxiety. Their emotional experience wasn't on my radar earlier. They were splendidly caring and compassionate, but now I could also see they were troubled. Consequently, there was a lot of nervous laughter that morphed into teasing me, one of my children's favorite activities. In the present circumstance, the ribbing injected a measure of normalcy. Soon we learned my surgery wouldn't start until the early afternoon.

Sarah fired off her first CaringBridge entry of the day during our wait.

> We're told Bret's surgery has begun and "is going smoothly." Very thankful for that update.

The Baldaufs are still hanging out and waiting to get the call from Dad's operating room and surgeon that it's time for him to roll that way. He's still sleepy from the drugs he got for the central-line procedure and feeling good and drowsy. Mom knew to ask for blankets from the warmer, so he's cozied up under some toasty covers.

A few hours ago, I went with Bret to pre-op and stayed there until his parents arrived. They're two very sweet, very kind people. Right now they're in the waiting room and my dad's sister, Roseann, is with them.

Bret was confident, clear-eyed, and upbeat this morning. In fact, as Emily, he, and I drove to the hospital he was scanning for good tunes on the radio. We all ended up singing and doing a little seat dancing to Rick James's "Super Freak." . . . So we're gathering all kinds of fun memories through this experience. ☺

xoxo to all—Sarah

Dr. Becker arrived around eleven thirty. She was calm and reassuring. Her review of the process was basically wasted on me because I was either unable or unwilling to focus on the details of what would happen. At this point I trusted her unequivocally. I was, however, glad the kids were there to hear it. Their better understanding of what was involved in transplant surgery helped me let go of responsibility, real or perceived. We tried our best to keep them updated and informed, but we probably didn't do justice to the medical procedures. To my recollection, all three asked questions, hopefully allaying their fears and shoring up their knowledge of what would transpire. Emily was rational and businesslike in her approach. Luke was quieter, bordering on stoic. Being the youngest of the three, Luke seemed slightly more reticent. Sarah, then a medical editor at *U.S. News &World Report*, had invested considerable time studying transplant procedures and was particularly disciplined and methodical. She approached Becker and my transplant as if she were covering it for the magazine.

In the waning minutes, floating through the final steps to surgery, I jettisoned any residue of effort to influence what was about to happen. To the extent possible, I was thoroughly immersed in the moment at hand. The last vestiges of conscious control were abandoned. Although being informed and active in my care was previously so important to me, as I laid there on the gurney, control and information were of absolutely no value whatsoever. It was perfectly OK to surrender and let the people who cared for me drive the bus and let the medical experts successfully do their thing.

In retrospect after processing this event, I realized I was shifting my approach to living. I had to adapt; my old beliefs and assumptions about maintaining control were challenged, and I had to change. This watershed health event necessitated those insights and awareness, but aging pushed me toward the same revelation. Our culture reveres strength and power, and as we age, our strengths and various capacities naturally diminish. We lose a step or two. Rationally, there's no shame in that, but we're culturally conditioned to resist and pretend the changes aren't occurring. Finding myself in such a formidable situation with few available options, I was forced to readjust my attitudes. For me, the attitudinal change that started that day was slow and filled with missteps, mistakes, and regressions. But persistence pays off in the long run. Integrating and accepting my losses, weaknesses, and vulnerabilities were other gifts of this difficult process.

With her tasks completed and her reassurances given, Becker departed to prepare herself for surgery. I vaguely recall her saying she might eat a bit before the surgery party started. I remember smiling to myself about how ordinary and even mundane my surgery was to her. The irony, even in my dopey state of mind, wasn't lost on me. I was about to have the most threatening and dangerous experience of my life, and Becker was going to have lunch. Life is life—beautiful, complex, filled with irony, and always happening on innumerable levels. Why would it be any different that day?

The transport tech arrived with his chariot to fly me to the pre-op area. This little ride was just like the ones you see on television shows. We wound down the halls, narrowly averting collisions because of the transport tech's expert skills. We arrived at the two large automatic doors that separated the ordinary routines of life from the sites of surgical interventions that might cure or restore. I knew the moment was at hand. The room was packed with doctors, nurses, and countless other medical personnel. I expected something statelier; it was like a subway terminal. Parked in a curtained-off area, the assault of interviews began. First the nurses, then a doctor, then an anesthesiologist, and finally a nurse anesthetist that Audrey had helped train and had worked with ten years earlier. All of them eagerly wanted to ask me something or perform a procedure. Perhaps the most essential part of what was about to happen had already been resolved. It was good to live with people in the medical business; Audrey prearranged who my nurse anesthetist would be beforehand and confirmed what drugs would be used. Any fears I had about being put to sleep were eliminated. Everyone was more than competent, friendly, and helpful. Everything humanly possible was done to reassure me that my surgery would be successful.

With only a few moments left before la-la land, I said farewell to each of the kids. One by one they gave me a hug, and we said to each other, "I love you." Never were those words more appreciated than in those last minutes before I was wheeled off to get another person's kidney. The intensity was palpable. Audrey lingered, and we had a *moment* in that minute. Never had I felt the power of being loved so intensely as in those fleeting seconds. Knowing my family loved me was more comforting than anything the doctors said or did. I felt peaceful and calm. Bring it on.

KIDNEY TRANSPLANTS

According to the Organ Procurement and Transplantation Network (OPTN), 16,815 transplants were performed in 2011, the year of my kidney transplant. Living donors accounted for 5,772 of those transplants—and Bret was one of those courageous donors. 11,043 were from deceased donors. Between January 1, 1988, and May 31, 2014, a total of 358,124 kidney transplants were performed.

The National Kidney Foundation reports that as of September 8, 2014, there were 123,175 people waiting for lifesaving organ transplants in the United States. Of these, 101,170 await kidney transplants. In 2013, 16,896 kidney transplants took place in the United States. Of these, 11,163 came from deceased donors and 5,733 came from living donors (a gain of only one living donor in two years).

Furthermore, by September 2014, the National Kidney Foundation states that, on average, three thousand new patients are added to kidney waiting lists each year. On average, twelve people die each day while waiting for a lifesaving kidney transplant. In 2013, 4,453 patients died while awaiting a transplant.

Based on statistics from 2013, of 4,715 living donors, only 462 came from unrelated paired donation and just one from an unrelated anonymous donation. All the other donations were from family members or spouses. So despite the wonderful, heartwarming stories you hear about strangers donating a kidney to a needy recipient, unrelated kidney donation is still relatively rare—0.098 percent.

There is a tremendous need for not only better education and understanding of being a donor, living and dead; but much needed improvement to how organs are procured from the deceased.

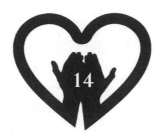

THE KINDEST CUT OF ALL

*Life can only be understood backwards; but it
must be lived forwards.*

—Søren Kierkegaard

My head was floating, and the rest of me with it. The word *subdued* best describes how I felt. The drugs worked perfectly. Swiftly and efficiently, the OR staff took over. I last saw Audrey standing by the exit door of pre-op as they wheeled me away. She looked lovely, worried, and frightened. I took comfort knowing that I never loved her more and was filled with gratitude for everything she'd done. With an assist from the potent drugs running through my veins, calm engulfed my entire being. I knew the situation was entirely out of my hands. Fear had disappeared. I was soothed by the knowledge that I'd done everything possible to get to this point. I hovered on the edge, about to jump off the cliff just like in the movie *The Abyss*—the difference being that I steadfastly believed my leap wasn't a one-way journey. I would return to those who loved and cared about me . . . with a chance for renewal. The odds were excellent that my body would be regenerated. There was no guarantee, but there were reasons for optimism.

In those last few moments, even in my cloudy, medicated state of mind, I realized that the Great Spirit, Yahweh, fate, God, Allah, Dr. Becker, chance, luck, or medical science (or perhaps all of them) were now in charge—anyone and anything but me. After being wound tight for the past eleven months, I welcomed letting go and having someone or something else take over. Other than a similar medical situation or in a catastrophic circumstance—like being on the deck of the *Titanic* or on a plane you know is going down—my situation might be the only time a person can truly, literally surrender. It was time to capitulate. It is strange how we frantic, fragile human beings bear the constant burden and strain of life almost all the time. Very seldom, if ever, do we get a reprieve from the encumbrances of living. The rare chance for freedom—a total release of responsibility and control—was at hand. With my physical body being watched over by medical experts, I surrendered.

A vivid memory of being wheeled into the operating theater and placed on the table remains to this day. We crashed through the double doors and a multitude of nurses, doctors, and techs flocked to me and lifted me from the gurney to the table. The room was cold and the commotion noteworthy. *Audrey lives in this world every day of her work life. Incredible! How does she manage?* As my last few seconds of awareness faded, I thought, *I hope you're on your game today, Dr. Becker.* Then everything went blank.

At 2:24 p.m. Audrey posted another CaringBridge entry, "It's Happening."

> Just got the call from the OR, Greg's surgery just started. They think they'll be getting Bret's kidney in less than an hour. Both of our guys are stable, and all is going well.
>
> Bret's parents, Al and Mary Lynn, are wonderful people. We all agree that it feels like we're family now, and that we've all known each other forever. Strange and amazing how the gift of Bret's kidney to

Greg has given exponentially to all of us.
Much love to all!
PS: The doc told us Greg has "pristine"
vasculature, which will help make his surgery
go swiftly. One of the many lessons in all of this:
exercise like Greg. It matters.

What transpired over the next three hours was reported to me later piece by piece. Audrey headed to the surgical waiting room where Sarah, Emily, Luke, Roseann, Bret's parents, and our friends Alan and Patty Rubin and Bernie and Susan Silver were waiting. I gather the situation was intense. Worry and laughter took turns. Anxiety battled optimism and hope. Resolve won. I never got the sense that any member of our immediate circle ever seriously thought I wouldn't make it through surgery. This prevailing attitude was a function of Audrey's experience in the OR and of how the kids "read" my position. With Luke leading the way, I had heard from each of them those past few days and months that they were taking their lead from me: if I was OK, so were they.

When I point-blank asked Audrey weeks earlier if I should be worried about the surgery itself, she responded, "There's always some risk. But I'm positive you'll wake up from the transplant procedure." I took enormous comfort in her perspective, not only because it was what I wanted to hear, but also because it seemed realistic, accurate, and based on her years of experience. When I asked Luke if he was worried about me, he said, "I'm not worried because you don't seem to be. I'm following your lead." Sarah, Emily, and Luke's attitude evolved because they trusted us. My refrain for years had been that I would keep them informed about my PKD and let them know when to worry or be afraid.

During the height of the surgical drama, Sarah and Emily both decided to post on CaringBridge.

Sarah added another CaringBridge entry, "Kidney Is in the Room."

Just got the call from the OR.

Bret's kidney has arrived in Dad's room.

This is about as real as it gets.

It should take several more hours for Dad's surgery to be done. Bret will be finished pretty soon, we hear—though in doctor speak, that could mean anything.

It took quite a few hours for the surgeon to get Bret's kidney, because the dude is so muscular. They're also very precise in their approach. All positive things.

We're in the waiting room with Bret's parents. Moments pass, sometimes with tears, sometimes with belly laughs. The gift Bret has given is overwhelming in its enormity.

Bret has shrugged off the thank-yous throughout the whole process. To him, this decision was a no-brainer. If there's anyone to thank, he has said, it's his parents. They taught him, he explains, that if someone is in need and you can do something to help, just do. Wow.

Audrey later shared that she had a mini breakdown in the waiting room. Audrey isn't overly emotional, particularly in a crunch. Among her strengths are her down-to-earth pragmatism, doggedness, and coolness in a crisis. Even though she might be churning on the inside, outwardly she is resolute and calm. Obviously, her coping style was reinforced by navigating the life-and-death situations she worked in every day, but it's also an integral part of her personality. That said, at one point during the ordeal of waiting, she had an encounter with Bret's mom, Mary Lynn. As Audrey tells it, she went to give Mary Lynn a hug to comfort her and she wound up completely breaking down, to the point of sobbing. Although uncharacteristic, Audrey's collapse was long overdue. Having withstood eleven months of living in disaster mode and being forced to be the strong one not only for me but also for the kids, Audrey was at her wit's end. I was relieved when I heard about it, hoping her waiting-room meltdown might prevent an even more severe breakdown later. During Audrey's emotional collapse, my friend Bernie walked in on the two women embracing and Audrey crying. He immediately thought I had died on the table and that was the reason Audrey was hysterical. All were relieved (me included) to hear that news of my demise was premature.

Considering none of us had met Bret's parents until that morning, there was a lot to say. Al and Mary Lynn Williams amused and perhaps shocked those present with stories about Bret as a young, restless boy growing up in Ohio. My favorite waiting-room story was when Al, Bret's dad, asked him to shovel the newly fallen snow on the driveway. Bret and his younger brother filled a large, two-handed squirt gun called a Super Soaker with gasoline, used it as flamethrower, and melted the snow to avoid shoveling it. Clever? Yes. Dangerous? Yes. Bret avoiding being burned or something worse was probably not the first or only time he'd put himself in harm's way. This firsthand account of Bret's wild streak gave context to a comment he'd made to me about his kidney doing better in me than him. (Spoiler alert: his kidney, now residing in me, hasn't displayed the same tendency toward risk-taking or rowdiness.)

With emotions running high, those in attendance tried to stay busy chatting and doing menial things to keep their minds off the situation. My sister, a two-time donor candidate, was her typical gregarious self. She probably wouldn't admit it, but Roseann, who's a fast talker to begin with, goes to warp speed in situations like this. Audrey confessed to me later that she was delighted my sister had engaged Bret's parents so she could sit quietly by herself (her natural coping style) or at least not feel she needed to take care of everyone.

Emily also used CaringBridge to post her version of what was transpiring. She called the entry "Close 'Em Up."

Just received an update that Bret is in recovery and doing well. It's been a long day already, but everything seems to be moving in the right direction. It has been a pleasure getting to know Bret's kind and loving parents. It's no wonder where he gets his generous and youthful spirit. They'll get to see their son shortly when he wakes up.

The traveling kidney has made it into our dad, Greg, who couldn't be more deserving of this amazing gift. He has always told us that the key to making it through these challenging times is to laugh and cry with your family and friends. Well, Pops, we've been doing both as we've shared the stories of these last few months. As I write this, we received word that Bret's kidney is now functioning in Dad, and they're starting to close him up. In my lovely sister's words, "I've never been so excited to hear he's producing urine."

Thank you all for your positive energy, thoughts, and prayers that have helped get us to this moment.

—Em

Sarah, the journalist and writer, spent her time as head blogger, updating the CaringBridge website with Audrey and Emily's help. My family reported that in those early days friends and family were unable to work because they were keeping up with the blog. Little did any of us know when we started blogging that Sarah's postings would create an incredible following that waited for the hourly entries from her or someone else. All of us were moved by the genuine caring, compassion, and support shown by so many wonderful people, some of whom I didn't even know. CaringBridge allowed Bret to be acknowledged for being the hero he truly was. People poured their hearts out in support of the man of the hour. The recognition for Bret brought me to tears every morning when Audrey or one of the kids read me the night's postings.

The most amazing benefit of the time around the surgery was that Audrey was taken care of by all three kids, especially her daughters. Each in their own way acted with remarkable love and care. We often talked about this role reversal that I think so few parents get to see. Having spent most of our adult lives as caretakers, like most parents do, we were moved by their ability to be adults when the situation demanded. We were never prouder of them.

Regular phone calls from the nurse in the operating room kept everyone updated on my progress. This progressive practice by the UChicago hospital was positive and very comforting to all present. Some of the group's favorite updates, I learned, were descriptions of Dr. Becker carrying Bret's kidney between operating rooms and, a little later, after the kidney had been transplanted, declaring that the kidney was "making urine." It was funny how a basic bodily function was vital to life at this moment.

One of the OR calls threw Audrey into a panic. Prior to surgery, we were told it would take four to six hours. With this information in mind, everyone hunkered down for a long, exhausting wait. When the phone rang again two and a half hours into the surgery, Audrey freaked for a second, feeling abject fear. Believing the surgery was hardly to the halfway point, she immediately thought something went terribly wrong. Did the procedure have to be terminated? In actuality, the nurse was calling to report, "They're all done." Even wonderful and extremely positive news could trigger fears of the worst-case scenario, demonstrating how fragile and emotional everyone was. Despite how well things went, coping was a challenge that afternoon. Frankly, I'm glad I wasn't there to witness it. Caretakers can have more stress and experience as much, if not more, emotional vulnerability as the patient.

At 5:07 p.m. Sarah wrote "A Smiling Surgeon" in CaringBridge:

We just had a glorious visit from Dr. Yolanda Becker, Dad's surgeon.

"It's a great kidney," were her words exactly.

She was smiling wide and explained the surgery went very well *and* that Dad had already produced 250 ccs of urine. Apologies for the graphic details, but this is the currency of a successful kidney transplant. (At this stage of the game, at least). Woo-hoo! Dad's surgery lasted less than three hours, which is excellent.

Bret, superhuman that he is, is in the recovery room. His first question: How's Greg? His goal is to walk from his recovery room down to the ICU where Dad will be tonight. If anyone can saunter down a long hallway hours after donating a kidney, I suspect Bret can.

We've truly had a joyous time hanging out in the waiting room with Bret's parents, Dad's sister, Roseann, and friends Patty and Alan Rubin and Bernie and Susan Silver. The laughs have gotten louder and the sighs of relief lighter as the good news has come in from Bret's and Greg's surgical teams.

Bret's parents can see him in about an hour. We'll probably have to wait an hour or two before we can see Dad in the ICU.

Until then we're basking in the delight of two successful surgeries.

I had survived surgery—just as I knew I would. Never a doubt.

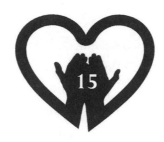

RENAL FAILURE IN THE
REARVIEW MIRROR

They say miracles are past.

—WILLIAM SHAKESPEARE

Still under the influence of powerful narcotics, when I arrived at the ICU I was woozy, unfocused, and drifting in and out of pseudo-awareness. It was weird—the lights were too bright, bordering on oppressive, and a plethora of medicos were observing me with very concerned, caring looks. Much to my surprise, there was no pain, largely because of the anesthesia still in my system from the surgery. Despite the grogginess, I was acutely aware that I was *alive*. Becker's and Audrey's prophecies were true—I survived the transplant surgery. I was ecstatic, but I couldn't express it. A partially drug-induced, but nonetheless real, bliss engulfed me. I was on the other side. The renal failure and debilitating kidney disease that dominated my life for the past eleven months were in retreat. I was now a kidney transplant patient and would be one for the rest of my life. The curse of managing a degenerative disease was no longer the overriding concern. Recovery was. I was thrilled about my new condition even before it was validated medically and before knowing what really happened in surgery. Things were changing fast. Someone or something had pushed the accelerator to the floor. *Hang on,* I mused to myself. *Things are about to get even more interesting.*

My reverie was abruptly interrupted by a harsh dose of reality. I was rolled into a private room, the gurney positioned next to a waiting hospital bed. The worried and determined look in Audrey's eyes betrayed her hypervigilance. She was on familiar turf. She switched from the role of spouse to being a nurse anesthetist, a highly skilled professional who had personally cared for hundreds of patients immediately after surgery. I sensed her nursing instincts kick in and took solace in it. She wouldn't allow anyone to screw up on her watch. I smiled to myself. I pitied the fool who stepped out of line.

The medical troops circled around to move me into the hospital bed. I was too drugged to do anything but passively let providence take over. As they started to lift me, my serenity, calm, and pain-free state abruptly ended. *Was that crazy witch doctor from* Indiana Jones and the Temple of Doom *ripping out my new kidney with his bare hand?* It felt like my gut was going to burst and my new kidney and intestines were going to fall out. Being lifted was agonizing. I wondered if they'd even bothered to sew me back up. Had they decided to save on sutures? After what seemed like an eternity of jostling, pushing, and shoving, I landed on the bed, my new home for the next couple of days. I dared not move. I lay very, very still as the pain lessened slightly. No more idle ruminations. Breathing was all I could do to calm down and subdue the nerve endings at the incision site.

Seeing me suffering, Audrey kicked into gear. She insisted the ICU nurse give me more Dilaudid, a synthetic heroin and my favorite narcotic whenever I was in the hospital. The nurse was reluctant to respond, saying she could start the new pain-management regimen as soon as she got my monitors hooked up, which would take far too long from Audrey's perspective. She knew the sooner the better to effectively curtail pain. After urging and then pestering, the nurse succumbed and agreed to contact the doctor on call so I could get an IV injection of the painkiller. The injection helped, but Audrey was still very frustrated that I had experienced this level of pain. She felt it could have been resolved by the nurse anesthetist before I left the OR. Be that as it may, the pain slowly subsided. Things were calming down.

At 6:17 p.m. that evening, as we all recovered, Audrey recorded the following CaringBridge entry:

> "I feel like I've been hit by a TRUCK."
> Those words just came out of Greg's mouth. We're in the ICU, and the truck's name was Dr. Yolanda Becker. Greg's anesthesia team stopped by and reported that the surgery was a "chip shot" that couldn't have gone smoother or easier, for both our boys. Pain is getting under control and Greg is doing well. Keep the good vibes coming. What a day!

Sarah quickly added:

> "He's peeing like a racehorse."
> That's what the nurse anesthetist, David Clanton, just came down to tell us.
> He also said we could go up to the ICU to see him . . . . ☺

After a brief ICU visit from the kids, Audrey and I were alone in the waning minutes of the most incredible, transformative day of my life. My courageous and committed wife was spent, but she offered to spend the night. After some "discussion," she agreed to go to the nearby hotel to at least rest and maybe even sleep. She felt pushed and pulled by her choice. But with the long ordeal of my recovery only beginning, she had to shut down, at least for a while.

Audrey's last entry of the day, "Signing Off for the Night," was posted at 10:25 p.m.:

What a life-altering day it's been for all of us.

Greg has been chatting with us here in his ICU room and his pain is way, way down. He's waxing and waning between being deeply humbled and goofy ol' Greg. The nurses and docs keep telling him how rockin' his urine output is. Greg wants to know if he'll win a prize. ☺

Bret looks great and is resting up. No trip from his room to Greg's today, but we'll have something to look forward to tomorrow.

Feels like we've been here for weeks, yet it's only been fourteen hours. Strangely, hospitals are kind of like casinos.

See you tomorrow. Thank you all for such wonderful, helpful, and sweet notes of encouragement. They mean the world to us all to know you're sending big love this way.

After Audrey left, I lay there in the hospital bed more awake than I wanted to be. Most of the pain was gone. My wakefulness was due in large part to the 500 milligrams of steroids I'd been given during the surgery. Straight ahead of me on the wall was a giant clock, like the ones in classrooms all around the country. I found myself staring at it. It seemed significant. I left one time zone and moved to another. More time was given to me. I was elated and pleasantly surprised to have reached this point. My "new" reality and time were beginning. I survived the surgery. A perfect kidney was functioning superbly in my body. My life had changed dramatically in the last few hours. A new resolve was forming in me to move forward into the future given to me. The most treacherous part of my adventure was over. I had just experienced a miracle, which was awe-inspiring. In those moments, no logic or reason could supplant these feelings of amazement, wonder, and humility. Time was no longer an enemy, but once again an ally and a gift.

Any real, or peaceful, sleep was elusive. I was "jacked up on 'roids." I floated in a dreamy state, somewhere between slumber and awareness. Thankfully, after the trauma of the bed transfer, my pain was limited. Being pain-free was a relief, especially after feeling such agony earlier.

Waking the following morning, I realized I had the privilege of a private room. In those hours after the surgery, I was progressively mindful of my incredible good fortune—so many things had gone my way. As a transplant patient I couldn't have been luckier—starting with Bret giving me a "perfect" kidney. It seemed inconceivable that my hot streak would continue, but it did. During my recovery, I said that I had won the high-stakes lottery—the prize was a restored life, with quality of life thrown in as a bonus.

I still had so many questions about my good fortune. Pursuing the answers—then and later—was a huge part of the motivation for writing this book. But even in those early moments, I asked, *Why am I so lucky?* That was my first and most prominent question. Many people told me I deserved the incredible fortune I was experiencing. And although it's flattering to the ego to accept that idea—I believed "deserving it" was more of a romantic notion than a reality. Many far better human beings than I have had horrible things happen to them. Not for a minute did I think I was more deserving than anyone else. The fact that I had survived and later would thrive filled me with humility. As recovery progressed, other questions emerged. *Why did I do so well? How much has luck or randomness factored into it?* I'm not sure how to answer these queries. It is difficult to believe *all* my good fortune was random or that the stars simply aligned to make it true. I might subscribe to that explanation if my good fortune consisted of a few random or lucky events, but the "luck" that repeated itself regularly for almost two years prevents me from buying it completely. The mystery remains, the questions continue, and answers remain elusive.

In those early hours of recovery, it wasn't difficult to imagine myself as the luckiest person on earth. I was overcome with gratitude. My miracle began with finding Bret and culminated with getting his kidney. Lying there in the hospital bed, with "my" new kidney functioning perfectly, *fortunate* and *thankful* only began to describe how I was feeling. *Deeply grateful for a miracle* gets closer.

A NEW KIDNEY IN THE HOUSE

Thousands of candles can be lighted from a single candle, and the life of the candle will not be shortened. Happiness never decreases by being shared.

—Buddha

I had a game plan for my hospital stay: be a good patient but actively participate in my care. Just as I'd been in the search for a kidney, I wanted to be an advocate for myself and my recovery. Audrey agreed. She supported this strategy and intended to champion me as well. Waiting for her to arrive the day after the surgery, I tried to take it all in. How strange it was to be lying in a hospital bed and how especially peculiar to be in an ICU. But there I was—like it, or not. I did my best to adjust to my surroundings as the tempo of the ICU accelerated rapidly. The nurse assigned to me performed an endless list of tasks—checking monitors, preparing meds, making notes, etc.—to check my postsurgical condition.

My condition was stable. My newly acquired kidney was performing magnificently. The critical factor now was the kidney's ability to make urine, so the nurses checked the output hourly. So far, so good. I smugly smiled and repeated the nurse's words, "The catheter bag is brimming with urine."

More clarity became possible as I returned to a more conscious state. The influence of the surgery—the trauma and the copious amount of drugs—remained, but my lucidity improved. Or so I thought as I attempted to follow what was going on around me. My belief about how aware and alert I really was amused my family and friends. But in those early moments, I needed to believe I was able to track my current medical condition.

I looked forward to Audrey's arrival. Her help was always welcome, and her presence gave me solace. But for the moment, I was reasonably relaxed and trusted the nurses to know what they were doing. As I waited for Audrey, I decided I was going to make it. Was it blind optimism, foolishness, or denial? I wasn't sure, but one thing was clear from the professionals around me—I was doing well. We chose the UChicago Medical Center because we believe it's the best in our area, and they appeared to be proving that was true. I was an inside observer to the workings of modern medicine. *Quite impressive.* Counting my blessings was a good way to pass the time.

The parade of doctors was starting just as Audrey arrived. She wanted to hear their reports. There had been a brief and preliminary visit from a pack of residents the night before to make sure nothing serious was wrong. Now the principal players were about to arrive.

Before she left the hotel, Audrey had made the first CaringBridge entry of the day, "A Great Night," at 8:54 a.m.

> We're headed to the hospital and will report some
> firsthand info about both our guys. Thanks for all the
> support. I've not been on this side of the medical
> fence before and can tell you, the other side is better.
> *But* I feel good about how things are going, and your
> posts are fabulous. I've been reading them to Greg. He
> loves them, but it hurts to laugh (that's OK).

The responses to CaringBridge posts from Audrey, Sarah, and Emily had been rolling in. All those in the waiting room the day before were bolstered by the offerings of genuine care, prayers, and healing energy. The volume of responses amazed me. I expected to hear from family members and close friends, but I didn't expect the breadth and depth of the voices—friends of friends, friends of our children, coworkers, colleagues, former students, and even people I didn't know and people from my past joined the chorus. My "birth cousin," and actual second cousin, Cathy Jorgensen (born the day after me at the same hospital), who chose my same profession and had been Aunt Marge's kidney donor, added her support and concern from Japan. These songs of love were beautiful!

Hundreds of messages were entered in the CaringBridge Guestbook. I cried, and then sobbed, as Audrey read them to me. The compassion washed over me and created a beautiful chorus of support from new posts, a refrain that was repeated multiple times each day at the hospital and then continued for weeks at home. Each reading lifted me up and fed my spirit. Without a doubt, this compassion fueled my healing. Love has a way of doing that to a person.

The first medical visit that first morning after the surgery was from the anesthesiologist. He described how well everything went and complimented Becker's skill and efficiency. We knew about her expertise, but we never tired of hearing about it. He then gave me a wonderful, unexpected compliment. "You have 'pristine' vasculature," he said. Wow! How about that! Just shy of sixty years, I was overjoyed to hear my arteries were clean as a whistle. Dr. Nash had urged me to stay heart healthy. My exercise and eating habits had paid dividends. My return to health began with the anesthesiologist's praise.

Dr. Becker's star shined even brighter in those first hours. Almost everyone we encountered in and around the ICU, doctors and nurses alike, praised her. One nurse described her as a "stud," meant in the most flattering way, I'm sure. The medical staff praised Becker's superior surgical skills and for how she treated them. Whenever she was in the ICU, they reported, she acknowledged them and their work and frequently solicited their perspective and opinions on patients. No wonder they held her in such high esteem. I was sad when Becker's role in my journey was ending. Once postoperative care started in the Transplant Clinic, her job was complete.

Laura was my nurse that first day after the transplant. As a twenty-year veteran of the ICU, she was an excellent nurse who demonstrated a welcome no-nonsense, practical approach to patient care. She was relaxed in how she ran the room. Therefore, because I was doing so well, my family and friends were allowed to visit with little or no restriction. This is atypical for ICUs, but it worked extremely well for us. Laura was so good Audrey made it a point to write the hospital administrators, complimenting her service and skills.

The first day progressed smoothly with someone always sitting by my side. A natural rhythm evolved. Periodically, a time-out was announced for me to doze off and rest. The room quickly quieted and any and all action ceased. Audrey or the kids acted as a gatekeeper.

Upon my return to wakefulness, they read the entries that came rolling in from the CaringBridge Guestbook the day after the surgery. Bill and Irene's missive is first, and other representative examples follow:

> Hi to all at the UChicago Transplant Dept. We are looking at your photos together and reading messages from *sooooo* many of your family friends. You are loved!!! And deserve to be. Add us to the list of your fans and people who care about you and now Bret and his family, who have become our family too. Donors are heroes in the true sense of the word. Add Bret to the family's other donors, Cathy and Paul. Thank you for the gift that keeps on giving. We are so happy to know that both surgeries went well and will visualize Bret and Greg sharing surgery stories today. Not sure if Bret's surgery was laparoscopic or not. We'll get the details later when

we see you. In the meantime, rest and heal and know
you are in our thoughts and prayers.

Love, Bill and Irene

Jack Steinberg, our old friend from Portland, added, "Yesterday was
like watching a slow-motion miracle. It's getting better all the time!!"

Then Smokey and Elaine Daniels, our dear friends from Santa Fe,
joined the parade.

Here's one for Bret.

Man, you are a hero. It was great to meet you at
the wedding, so we could begin to understand
your courage and your character, and to enjoy your
humor and energy. (You were also the coolest guy in
the tent, so it was easy to spot you.)

You may have given up a kidney, but you have
gained an aunt and uncle in New Mexico who will
have your back forever. We hope you and Greg can
have that ceremonial scotch as soon as it's cleared by
the nurses!

To Bret's parents, what a fine son you have raised.

Love, Smokey and Elaine

Stacey Grisch, the wife of Audrey's nephew John Grisch, added:

Bret,

You are like a silent hero. I just want you to know
that someday I will tell my two boys about you when
they are old enough to understand. Granted one
is only three months and the other three years old
but I will tell them this story. It is a teaching story
of generosity, courage and incredible kindness. We
need more men in this world like you.

God bless, Stacey

My cousin Ken, one of my would-be donors, wrote:

> Greg and Bret,
>
> You are both heroes in my book! Stay strong, and feel
> the love and support of all these friends, family, and
> even strangers, as I am too. Bret, life is precious, and
> the gift of life is even more so. Keep on keepin' on!
>
> Ken B.

The CaringBridge posts sustained me on so many levels throughout my struggles. The words people shared were a beautiful and ongoing part of the compassion I was basking in immediately after surgery.

My relatively pain-free condition changed with a visit from the physical therapists—two hulking linebackers who played for the Chicago Bears. Or perhaps they were two Orcs that escaped from Middle-earth and cleverly disguised themselves as attractive, young female professionals. The nursing staff announced their impending visit throughout the morning, saying they would teach me how to get out of the hospital bed. If not for my muddled state, I would've realized they were warning me to hide. The therapists' mission: coerce me to get up and sit in a chair for twenty to thirty minutes that day and then repeat every following day, increasing in frequency and length. Getting up hurt like hell. Even though they urged me to press the morphine drip button to reduce the impending pain, I wasn't prepared for the shift from comfort to agony. I might have even pleaded, "Be merciful." But the physical therapists couldn't be dissuaded from their task. Much to my chagrin, up I got. Moving caused excruciating pain! I thought I would damage my fragile abdomen or open the stiches. In response to the well-meaning coercion, I repeated this act a few more times. Only later did I feel a sense of accomplishment.

As the activities slowed, my thoughts turned to Bret. I hadn't thanked him since before the surgery. I received regular reports about him, but neither of us could walk the few hundred yards to visit. Just then, walking down the hall seemed as Herculean a task as traversing a glacier. The donor frequently has a worse recovery than the recipient. Regrettably, Bret was no exception. He was in a lot of pain. The kidney was removed with Bret inverted and injected with large amounts of carbon dioxide to make the extraction easier, causing him to become bloated. Because Bret was so muscular, he retained the carbon dioxide. Consequently, his symptoms were like a case of the bends, the condition divers experience if they surface from deep water too quickly. Thousands of air bubbles in his muscle tissue were popping like cellophane bubbles, creating lots of suffering. Bret refused to take any pain medication and relief wasn't available through other medical means. Sarah, Emily, Luke, and Terry made sure he wasn't alone, and laughter helped heal his pain. I was proud and relieved that they took care of him.

Sarah made a CaringBridge entry around 2:26 p.m. on Thursday:

> Let the healing begin! . . . But nobody said it would be easy or fun.
>
> Good news to report. Bret and Dad have both gotten up out of their respective beds and are each spending time sitting up. This is a big deal. Both of them will be spending more and more time in a chair each day, eventually working up to walking. Strolling may happen today, maybe tomorrow. But those boys will walk.
>
> The reality is that Bret is feeling the brunt end of the surgery stick right now. He had a long surgery, is way muscular, and had a number of abdominal incisions. Of course, he's also adjusting to having one kidney instead of two. Very, very thankfully, he's starting to catch some sleep this afternoon.
>
> This morning, Dad was pleased to see the cadre of attractive physical therapists come into the room, but later referred to them as "little fascists" after they wouldn't let him cheat getting out of bed ("No

elevated bed for you!"). Dad said this smilingly, lovingly, and with a laugh, of course—and after they'd left the room.

Enough of the urine talk. Let's move on to a new measure of success: creatinine levels. We all have this measured with typical blood work, and it's critical to watch in kidney disease. Right before Emily's wedding on October 1, his went up to 7.6, which meant he was headed directly for dialysis and in full-on kidney failure (this technically happened earlier, but the severity increased significantly). Normal is between 1 and 2. But because of Bret's kidney, Dad's creatinine is already down to 3.3—that's in just a matter of hours. This, too, is big, big, BIG news.

And finally . . . Bret's parents were able to come up to the ICU to meet Dad. Needless to say, hearing him say quietly and tearfully to Al and Mary Lynn, "Your son saved my life—I don't know how I'll ever thank him" . . . was powerful, surreal, and magical. Just as much, it was such a sweet and loving response.

As my first full day with a new kidney wound down, I was spent, and I looked like hell. Even though the day went exceptionally well, I wasn't out of danger. Still, there were no immediate causes for concern. Medically, my recovery progressed as well as could be expected. I was calm, resolute, and sustained by gratitude. I wanted to get better as quickly as possible.

As darkness fell, Audrey and I agreed it would be a good idea for her to return to Evanston. Going home to our bed increased the odds of her sleeping. I was in good hands. Shortly after her exit around ten o'clock, I was given sleep medication. My steroid dose was reduced, but sleep was still a challenge. I dozed off, relishing that I'd survived day one. I felt myself moving from *surviving* toward *healing*. The first two major steps on my journey to a new life—getting a donor and having the transplant—were realized. All I had to do now was recover.

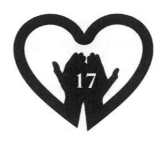

WHIZZING ALONG

The routine of day two initially resembled day one; it was filled with hustle and bustle. Nurses scurried around as they checked various monitors, and the phlebotomist drew blood from the IV site in my arm. Of the four intravenous lines in me, two were in use, and the other two were backup sites in case of an emergency. They reminded me of the seriousness of my predicament.

My pain continued to be minimal. The only time I pressed the patient-controlled analgesia (PCA) button was to sit up in the bedside chair. Being relatively pain-free encouraged optimism and lessened my concerns about recovery. The one discouraging circumstance was that Laura, our marvelous nurse from the day before, wasn't on duty. The quality of attention wasn't diminished, but the younger nurses were more rigid in their approach to patient care and far stricter about allowing visitors access. We were reprimanded for having too many people in the room. Consequently, as the day passed, a tension developed between us and the nursing staff—resulting in them avoiding us at times when we thought they might have been more helpful.

During the morning activities, I couldn't wait for Audrey, Sarah, Emily, and Luke to arrive. I longed for the emotional safety they brought. When they arrived, we settled down to read from the CaringBridge blog. Without fail, halfway through the first one, I started to cry and didn't stop until the last one. Who knew it was possible for words to be so powerful? My physical healing was covered by excellent medical care, and the love expressed by my family and friends was healing my spirit. This response from my cousin Sharon illustrates the tone of the posts:

> Welcome to the club, gentlemen!
>
> Bret, you have now joined Paul and Cathy as superheroes for our family. There is no greater gift than life. Thanks, thanks, and thanks forever!
>
> Greg, now the big challenge (once you get used to all the meds): how do you pay it forward? Life is now changed for you forever. How lucky can we get?
>
> Yay to the great transplant team and the researchers behind the scenes. Soon PKD will be a thing of the past. We'll freeze the Freese gene (where PKD originated in our family) in time.
>
> With you in spirit, and sending you light and love. Celebrate daily!

After the reading of the posts ended and our emotions settled, Sarah updated the CaringBridge blog with an entry she titled "First Time in 40 Years."

> More amazing news: Dad's creatinine level is down to 1.4!
>
> I made a mistake yesterday when I wrote that the normal range is between 1 and 2. It's actually between 0.8 and 1.5, according to Dad's nurses. So the fact that Dad's is now within the normal range is

outstanding. He's not seen a result like that in forty years, circa 1971 when he was rocking long hair, insane facial hair, bell bottoms, and a big campus swagger at Southern Illinois University.

As his surgeon, Dr. Becker, said, "That kidney's going gangbusters."

Wahoo!

Later Sarah posted another note called "Everything Is Amplified."

Yesterday was rough for Bret. Really rough. But we've got some excellent signs that he's on the mend: He had a taste for a caramel macchiato (check), was amenable to a Potbelly roast beef sandwich (check), and has the energy for and interest in a little time on the computer (check). He's also making jokes and smiling again. We've been texting these small but significant updates to his parents. We all feel so connected in such a short, albeit intense, period of time. Once I head back to DC on Sunday, I may be compelled to start texting them updates about what my husband is eating and his general mood—I'm enjoying giving them the play-by-play so much.

It's been absolutely thrilling to see Bret's pain and demeanor improve. In this surreal world we're in right now, everything is so elemental, and the tiniest positive changes have brought enormous joy.

Friday was moving day: I was transferred to a different room in the ICU and later to a room on the hospital's surgical floor. Apparently, I was progressing well enough and without any complications. There were ample amounts of urine and the results of my blood tests, particularly the creatinine level, were excellent. In fact, my creatinine was 1.0. To put that in perspective, that creatinine result reflects the kidney function of people born with two perfect kidneys. Unbelievable! I hadn't experienced kidney function like this since I was a teenager. The kidney from Bret was working beautifully. *Hallelujah!*

Because she was attending a medical conference, I hadn't spoken to or seen Dr. Becker since the surgery. She followed my progress continuously with the ICU medical staff, the other surgeons on the transplant team, and the nephrologists. During one of those conversations with her colleagues, Becker introduced the possibility that I might be released from the hospital soon. By early Friday afternoon the ICU nurses were mentioning the possibility that I might go home on Saturday. *Is it even possible? Home three days after the transplant?* I was feeling good enough to want to get home, but I also feared leaving. But some of the events that transpired throughout the day would push me past my fear and hesitation.

About midday I transferred out of the individual room in ICU to a temporary ICU room until a bed was available on a surgical floor. We settled in as best we could, but the first hint of tranquility in the new space was interrupted by the physical therapists. Those lovely monsters were there to help me walk. I had no choice. It took forever to get me up and ready. All the wires and monitors had to be rearranged before I could take a step. The ability to walk was crucial; the sooner I sauntered, the sooner I got out. We took a stroll into the hall and circled the ICU. Pained and precarious as I was, I shuffled along. I had the "surgical stoop," the body's instinctive curving inward of the spine to protect the stomach and the large incision that covered most of it. I felt a hundred years old and acted like an invalid. I had to relearn the basic activity of putting one foot in front of the other. I walked, tearfully. I felt vulnerable and weak in new and uncomfortable ways. Little did I know then it would take months to regain my physical strength and learn to trust my body again.

Two noteworthy events occurred shortly after the change of venues. Both had an undeniable wow factor. First, Dr. James Chon, the head of the nephrology team in UChicago's Transplant Clinic, visited me. He was the nephrologist who had medically screened Bret and oversaw the process of him becoming a donor. Dr. Chon was protective of Bret, as he should have been. After chatting about how I was feeling, Dr. Chon told me something that will stay with me for the rest of my life. With tears in his eyes, he told me how fortunate I was to get Bret's kidney, adding that the kidney was "pristine." I had received a perfect organ. Dr. Chon went on to emphasize that I *must* take care of the gift I was given. His brief statement only confirmed what I already knew. But his words imprinted on my heart. In my experience, it's unusual for a physician to tear up when speaking to a patient, so Dr. Chon's heartfelt sincerity was stunning. Audrey and I looked at each other, acknowledging that a rare and significant moment had just transpired.

Awe and gratitude filled my heart, sending tremors through my entire being. I recognized the transcendence of this transaction between Bret and me. The enormous magnitude of Bret's gift was put into sharp relief by Dr. Chon's words. I wondered how to take it in, what to make of it, and how it would impact my life. The urge to share my story with others was growing stronger.

The other remarkable event that day was finally seeing Bret. He had recovered sufficiently from his battle with pain and was able to walk down to the ICU. The nurses granted reluctant permission for our entire family to be in the room at the same time. When he entered, my eyes filled with tears. It was a struggle not to break down completely. That my entire family—of which Bret was now an official member—was there to witness our reunion heightened the intensity of our emotional encounter. *This guy's a hero, and he doesn't even know it,* I thought. The room overflowed with wonder and gratitude. What a moment!

We chatted, laughed, and swapped war stories about what had happened to each of us. Bret was true to form; he fiercely wanted to get out of the hospital but remained stoic about it. He downplayed the importance of what he'd done. But I saw the tremendous kindness in his eyes and the depth of his soul that afternoon. Bret distinguished himself by his display of his giving, courage, and humility. I can't help but think most donors share similar attributes. I hope Bret can someday acknowledge what he did for me, and for our family. Until he does, we'll just have to keep working on convincing him.

Sarah completed the day's CaringBridge posts by sharing her perspective in an entry entitled "They Meet Again."

> Tonight, Bret walked over from his room to see Dad in the ICU.
>
> Emily, Terry, Luke, and I were hanging with Bret in his room joking around and laughing (painful for Bret, but good medicine nonetheless) when Bret decided it was past time to see Dad. The moment was go. And so we did.
>
> The five of us made the long walk—five corridors and four bends—from Bret's unit to the ICU. Bret pushed a wheelchair yet seemed to glide along pretty damn smoothly. If you saw him dancing at Emily and Terry's wedding, you know that he's got quite the moves, which his mother takes credit for, we learned. ☺
>
> So what do two guys—who now share tissue, an organ, and the gift of continued life—say to each other? Apparently, not a lot.
>
> Words just wouldn't have fit. Instead hands connected, eyes locked, jaws clenched, and tears welled.
>
> Of course, we women in the audience had tears streaming down our faces. But this moment was between two men. Bret and Dad. I'm not sure there will ever be proper words to convey the breadth of gratitude, emotion, or meaning surrounding this gift from Bret to Dad.
>
> I think that's OK. Sometimes you just know.

After Bret left, things slowed down. With the kids gone, Audrey and I faced the evening alone.

My inability to move my bowels loomed large and affected the possibly of going home the next day. Nothing helped in those early stages. I became, for the first time, irritable, short-tempered, and very uncomfortable. This unfortunate physical situation was coupled with the fact that now we were just marking time before going home. We had just touched the sky, and now we were wallowing in the mud. The only interruption that evening was when the ICU nurse removed the catheter. *Ouch.* Talk about your good times. Audrey was also in purgatory; she didn't want to leave me until the room change was made. She summoned her inner warrior and stayed the course.

The move out of the ICU at about nine o'clock that evening led to a series of unfortunate events that shaded our otherwise marvelous experience at the hospital. We were sent to a regular surgical floor close to Bret's room. By the time we left the ICU, no doubt everyone was glad to see us go. The ICU nurses, though professional to the end, weren't used to dealing with patients who were doing as well as I was, or who were accompanied by a private nurse. For all involved, this parting of the ways was a win-win.

Arriving on a surgical floor was a big change. There were fewer nurses so less attention would be paid. *Welcome to modern hospital care,* I thought. The room was extraordinarily hot and I roasted for a few hours before realizing the room had its own thermostat. Audrey was in a quandary. She didn't want to abandon me in my time of need, but she'd crossed her own threshold of tolerance and was slipping quickly into a state of exhaustion. At any other time seeing her in this pummeled condition would have sent me leaping into action to help her. But I was in no condition for a rescue. Tensions were running high; for the first time since I'd arrived at the hospital, it felt like we were faltering.

The most alarming threat arose over confusion about whether or not I had taken my steroid medication. It felt like a betrayal. I balked at taking another dose. I asked them to call the ICU to double-check. The ICU nurses said, "Ask him." We were at the low point in my treatment. Expecting me to track my medications in the hospital seemed totally preposterous. The hospital no longer felt safe, and Audrey and I were pissed. I wound up signing a form saying I refused my evening medication. My internal voice screamed, *Get me out of here!*

After the situation calmed down, we decided Audrey should leave, even though it was now eleven o'clock. I was concerned about her driving. Assuring me she could make it safely home, she left. I made her promise to call me when she arrived. Our parting words that night revolved around how much we wanted to get out of the hospital. Though not seriously in harm's way, I no longer felt secure. The fragile bond of trust had broken.

I was left with a simple but necessary task to accomplish my goal— have a bowel movement by noon tomorrow. Success was the only way out. After almost a year of immersion in the world of medicine, doctors, and hospitals that culminated in transplant surgery, it all came down to the most elementary task. My focus turned to suppositories and laxatives. I was hell-bent on accomplishing my task . . . tomorrow.

The room cooled, and, mercifully, I fell asleep. My last conscious thought that night: *Please take me home.* (Thank you, Phil Collins.)

In the wee hours of the morning, while I slept, a lovely CaringBridge entry was made by our friend, Margaret Hershey:

> So for those who haven't seen the picture of Greg
> and Bret seeing each other for the first time after
> the surgery—make sure you pull it up. This picture
> goes beyond "saying it all." Two guys/boys/men
> (of different generations) in the most vulnerable of
> positions; wearing hospital gowns, wrist bands, and
> huge smiles . . . and clasping each other's hands.
> It's beyond a miracle. Who would've thunk that
> some guy from Ohio—out of nowhere—would
> decide to give his kidney to someone he doesn't

even know? What are the chances??? How can we
not believe in the goodness of man/woman . . .
[and] the influence of parents who teach and model
values to their children.

Bret—don't be too modest. What you did was
heroic. I hope you can (at least a little bit) bask
in the glory and happiness of your unselfishness.
This picture could/should be the cover of *Time*,
Newsweek, *Ms.*, whatever. It emanates pure joy.
"The child is father to the man" comes to mind.
Sarah, Em, Audrey, Jerry, Smokey—you could
probably think of a better title. I also love the
juxtaposition of something so monumental taking
place concurrently with the everyday/ordinary, i.e.,
Em in the background, hand on hip, laughing as if
she's probably relating something from her wedding.
Such is life, huh? I'd like to have the picture, enlarge
it and place it somewhere I could see it every day,
to remind me of goodness, hope, miracles, and the
mundane and how they coexist in everyday life.

Apparently healing never sleeps.

GETTING OUT WHILE THE GETTING'S GOOD

My mission in life is not merely to survive, but to thrive;
and to do so with some passion, some compassion,
some humor, and some style.

—MAYA ANGELOU

Made possible by my superb nurse—a young Filipina woman whose name I unfortunately don't recall—I got some much-needed sleep that night. She was exquisitely dedicated, patient, and committed to do the right thing. She took the time to resolve the issues with my medication. This angel's conscientiousness wrestled victory as I slept. Medical technologies are marvelous, of course, but it takes human beings—nurses, technicians, and doctors—to invest the time and energy to make it all work. And she did. I was back on track after the room change and associated unpleasantness. This kind caregiver disguised as a nurse also had the human decency not to wake me in the middle of the night or early in the morning. She let me sleep. As Shakespeare put it, "Sleep that knits up the ravell'd sleeve of care."

On Saturday morning I was calmer and in a far better mood. I was "very likely" going home. The possibility of getting out of the hospital lifted my spirits, setting the tone for the day. After the usual tests, I summoned my strength to perform the main event: I took my stool softener and inserted the suppository. Then, for the first time in days, I ordered breakfast. I wasn't really hungry, but I was eager to normalize the situation. I wanted to feel regular. (Pun intended.) The food arrived; mediocre never tasted so good. With my attitude revitalized and my meal complete, I set my sights on getting out of the hospital. And it was only eight o'clock in the morning. I was on hospital time.

The plan was to rest and walk the hallways—ten minutes every hour or so would suffice. My first stop was Bret's room. He was talking to the doctor who performed his surgery and would authorize his release. We agreed to meet later. I focused on my other purpose. I desperately hoped walking would increase my peristalsis and lead to a bowel movement. It felt awkward roaming the halls. I was struggling, but I would've walked the twenty miles to Evanston from the UChicago hospital in the Hyde Park neighborhood in order to secure my release.

Bret was still moving gingerly as he came into my room. Abdominal surgery does that to a person, even when you're strong as he was. An awareness of how extraordinary he was to me and my family was fully present as I lay in the bed and he sat in a chair that morning. Our conversation was ordinary but heartening. There was no talk about the meaning of what had transpired between us. It was just two guys chatting. What was said was of little importance; being together was what mattered. He was coming home with us for a few days, and I welcomed spending some time with him in a more relaxed situation.

When Bret left, I sat for a while trying to take in what had happened over the last few days specifically and the last eleven months generally. I wanted to absorb the miracle, but not force its understanding. Being conscious and aware of it was sufficient for the moment. When my reverie ended, I set myself to the task at hand. I desperately wanted to do the deed before Audrey and the kids arrived. Pooping in the hospital that day ranked up there with the most painful and difficult things I did throughout my ordeal. Not quite as acutely painful as my initial move from the surgical gurney into the hospital bed, this was more of a persistent than acute pain. But I survived the final push, so to speak. Now get me home.

Audrey's arrival was joyous. She was my ticket out and, most importantly, my ally. My stark and undeniable dependency on her reminded me I couldn't do this alone. She too was adamant about leaving, arguably wanting me out of the hospital even more than I did. With her entire career spent working in them, she was acutely aware of the liability of staying in a hospital too long—mostly the possibility of iatrogenic infections, i.e., those acquired in the hospital itself. But more than any bacteria I might contract, the hospital no longer felt compatible or helpful to me. The rest of my recovery needed to be in the safer confines of my own home. I would sing the praises of everyone at the UChicago hospital for the rest of my days, but I desperately wanted out of there.

While we waited, Audrey read some of the posts. Among them was this note from Smokey:

> Those of us in the Santa Fe branch continue to be amazed by the boys' progress. Touched by their brotherhood, and inspired by the eloquence of the friends writing on this blog. Sarah, you should turn this story and these documents into a book that would not only be a best seller, it would illustrate the inherent goodness and altruism that Margaret H. so beautifully described a few posts back.

Having become regular again, four tasks remained: 1) Remove all the IV lines; 2) take out the central line, which would require a doctor; 3) sign the release papers; and 4) resolve the medication dosages. Simple, right? Audrey and I knew these modest chores could take hours. All in all, we worked through the list fairly smoothly until the final one. Confusion about the medications could sabotage our departure. The sheer number of pills I was required to take made me feel like I was on a forced outing to Pills "R" Me, a nightmarish version of Toys "R" Us. I received a parting gift—a large box from the pharmacy with all the necessities. Audrey checked my meds; she had familiarized herself with what I was taking. When the nurse reviewed the dosages, we knew immediately that something was wrong. The dosages she indicated had obvious errors. Looking at each other, we silently agreed to not say anything, knowing that unraveling the mistakes could take hours. We also knew we had backup—my first Transplant Clinic visit was early Monday morning. We only had to survive forty-eight hours on our own. We smiled, took the box, and made our getaway.

By this time the entire family was gathered in my room. We decided to depart in shifts: Bret (who already had his walking papers in hand) left first with Emily, Terry, and Luke. Audrey, Sarah, and I followed shortly thereafter. Sarah retrieved the car. With me in a wheelchair and Audrey by my side, we made our exit. As we traveled the corridors on our way out, a wave of anxiety hit me. Three and a half days after arriving, I was leaving with a new kidney. I was weak and unsure, and I felt extremely vulnerable, more so than I had ever felt or even imagined feeling. By the time we reached the car, the full import of reentering the world hit me. My emotions were all over the place. How was I going to manage, to heal? My incision felt like it might burst at any second. I hadn't felt this fragile since I was a child. But there I was—leaving the protective womb of the hospital. And determined to do so.

It felt like jumping off a cliff. The prospect was as engrossing as it was terrifying. My new future awaited, but first I had to make it through this transition. Leaving was the next proactive step in my healing and recovery. I needed to challenge myself and move beyond my limitations. The last few days dramatically changed what I thought

I knew. Along with the new kidney, my growing awareness was to be another life-altering gift. Sitting in the back seat waiting to depart, my emotions ran rampant: elation, apprehension, and fear. The steroids amplified my emotional lability. Thank god for Audrey and the kids. Without them, I would have melted, leaving a pool of raw emotions in my place.

All the way home, despite Sarah's skilled and cautious driving, vulnerability dominated. Each time she pressed the brakes to slow or change lanes, the incision burned. I was compromised physically. But the external world had little to do with my experience in those moments. Anxiety ruled my emotional experience and would for a long time to come. It led to my being irritable and crass. I became a "difficult" patient. Being ill-tempered was humbling, but it was inevitable.

When we pulled into the driveway and I put my feet on the ground, tears welled up in my eyes. The anxiety released. The tension—which had been persistent, intense, and overwhelming—rapidly dissipated. I was able to breathe again. I was home.

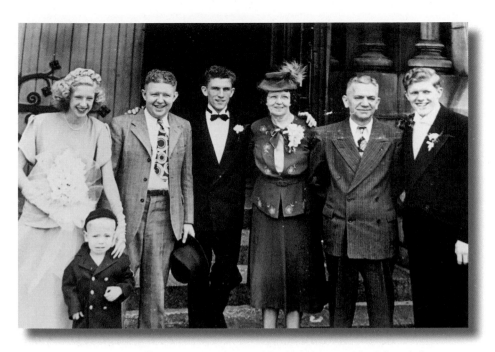

The origin of my PKD: my uncle Carl's wedding (1947). Pictured from left to right are my aunt Marge; my brother Jerry; my father George; my uncle Bill; my grandmother Ann; my grandfather Carl; and my uncle Carl. Ann was the carrier of the PKD gene. All of my father's siblings pictured here had PKD.

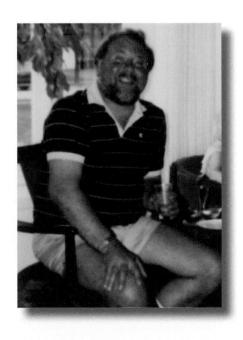

My brother Tom, approximately ten years after his transplant. You can see the effects of his medications, particularly the prednisone (steroid), which resulted in the puffiness of his appearance.

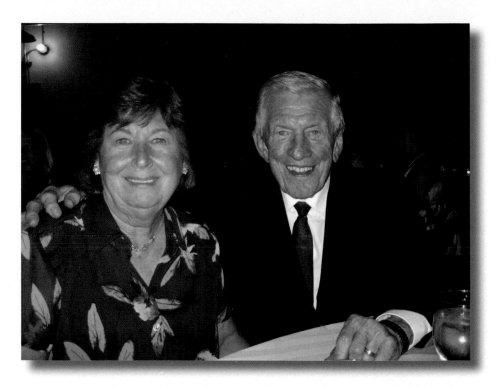

My uncle Bill and aunt Irene, the last members of their generation and the reigning patriarch and matriarch of our family. Bill and Irene were essential to my transplant success, showing love, support, and kindness throughout.

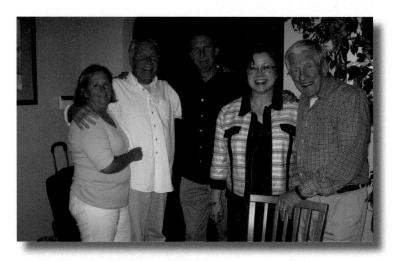

Dinner at our house after Ken's first day of medical tests at UChicago Hospital. Left to right: Audrey, me, Ken, Roseann, and Bill. Irene took the picture. Roseann and Ken together, my two heroes and would-be donors.

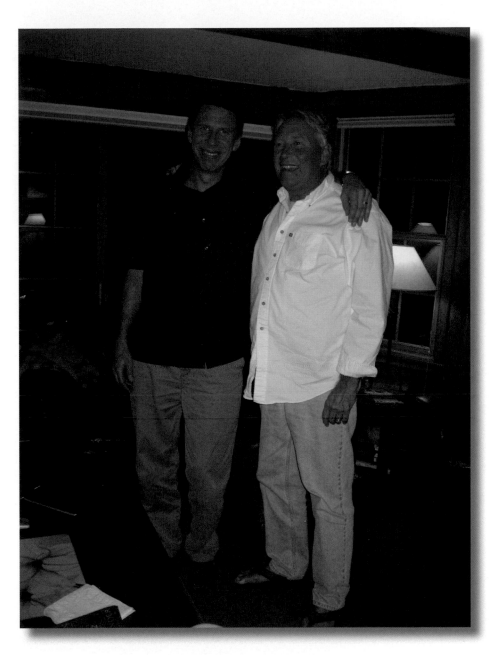

Ken and I, relaxing before dinner after his first day of testing.

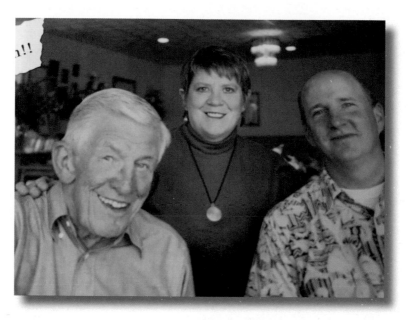

Bill, Sharon, and Paul May, her kidney donor. Sharon and Bill were instrumental in helping my kidney transplant story reach a glorious conclusion. Paul donating his kidney to Sharon convinced me success was possible.

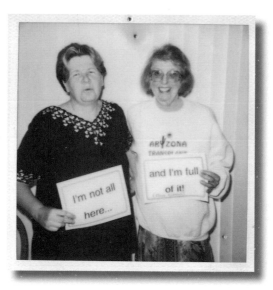

Aunt Marge, right, with her donor, Cathy Jorgensen,
my second cousin, on the left.

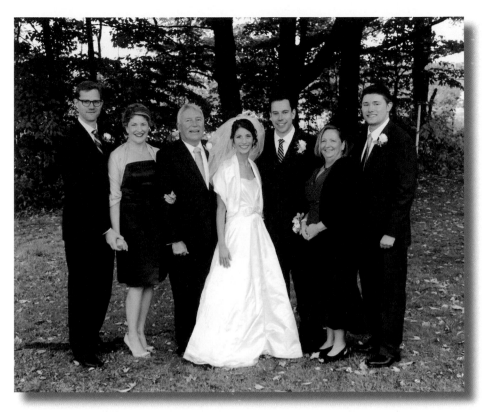

Emily's wedding picture of our family. This joyous event signaled that we'd made it to October 1. My transplant was only days away. Left to right: Chris, Sarah's husband; Sarah; me (looking a bit fragile); Emily, the effervescent bride; Terry, her new husband; Audrey; and Luke.

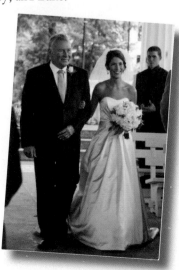

A happy memory of escorting Emily down the aisle.

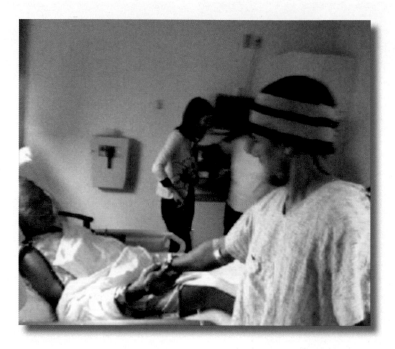

Bret's first successful visit to see me in the ICU after
a few failed attempts.

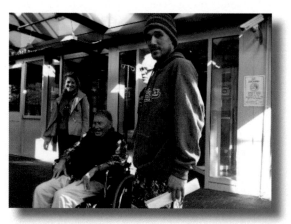

Sarah, Bret, and I wait for the car to take us home to
Evanston. I look scared and weak. Bret looks strong.
My new life was about to begin—ready or not!

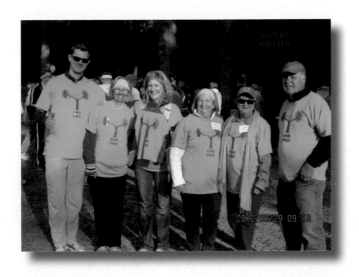

The Walk to End PKD that Emily organized, September 29, 2012. Left to right: Chris Fickes, our son-in-law; Beth Schabel, Emily and Terry's close friend; Sarah; Audrey; Maizie, Audrey's sister; and Bill, Maizie's husband.

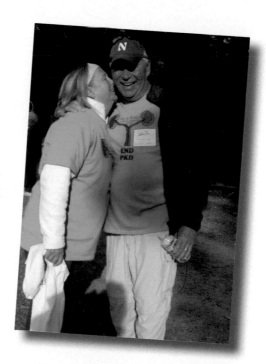

Audrey and me at the Walk to End PKD. My protruding stomach was not a side effect I was fond of.

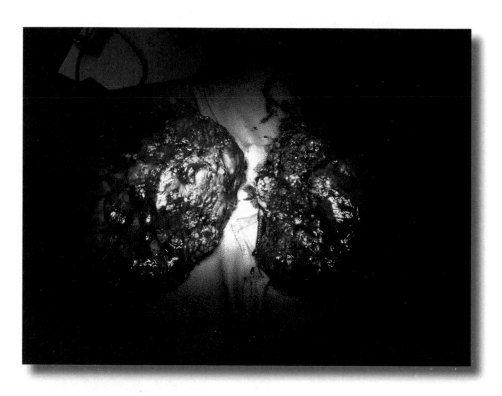

My polycystic kidneys: the culprits and the *why* of my story. On November 12, 2012, I had a double nephrectomy to remove my diseased kidneys. Dr. Tom Keeler, my urologist and assisting surgeon, took this photo in the OR.

HOME AGAIN, HOME AGAIN, RAT-A-TAT-TAT

Believe that life is worth living and your belief
will help create the fact.

—WILLIAM JAMES

For as long as I can remember, I've been breaking down tasks into parts. I learned this strategy from long-distance running—one mile, then two, and so forth. Deconstructing tasks makes them easier for me to complete. Now I could place mental checkmarks next to the first three items on my four-part list from months earlier: 1) Survive renal failure, 2) Find a donor, 3) Have transplant surgery, and 4) Recover and heal successfully. The third phase of my adventure was complete; I now possessed a new, twenty-seven-year-old, "perfect" kidney. As satisfying as success was, my remaining objectives—recover and heal—were formidable, and they loomed large on the horizon. A sense of accomplishment lingered for a time, but then faded. As I sat in my favorite chair—weak, depleted, and scared—I was reluctant to move. *Maybe,* I thought, *if I sit quietly and don't move, things will automatically reset to the way they were.* I longed for a break. *Enough is enough. Don't make me do anything else.* But underneath the inertia, I knew I was merely standing at a new starting line. *Ready. Set. Go!*

The whole family was with me, including Bret, now an "uber-official" member. Everyone was sweet, kind, and attentive. I felt loved to an infinite degree. Their comfort was a tremendous source of strength and motivation. I took it all in, letting it wash over me. It helped prepare me for my first effort and what I desired most—a shower.

I hadn't showered since Wednesday morning. Stewing in my own juices had reached its maximum level. *Ugh!* Two main hurdles stood between me and showering. I was weak and unable to stand for more than a few minutes, and I had a rather large, hockey-stick-shaped incision on my lower-right abdomen. I had expected it to be six to nine inches long; it was closer to twice that length. Thanks to Audrey's adroit application of a quasi-waterproof cover over the bandage, the second challenge was overcome. And the effort to shower was worth it. Even though I needed to lie down afterward, I felt rejuvenated. More than the sweat and hospital residue were expunged; I washed away eleven months of struggle, worry, and fear. I felt renewed and reborn. The simple acts of cleansing and purging were giant steps toward the new normal.

The real agony arrived when Audrey, nurse in residence, changed my dressing. Because my abdominal muscles had been cut, any movement was excruciatingly painful. (Abdominal surgery makes every muscle in your body feel directly connected to the incision.) Getting into or up from a reclined position was like someone pouring scalding-hot water on my stomach. Complementing this torture was the fear of splitting the stitches. To redress the wound, a cruelty required twice a day, I needed to be in a quasi-supine position, using about eight pillows to prop me up. It f*@#king hurt! It was weeks before the intensity of the pain of changing the dressing began to subside. No preparation could prevent the agony; it could only be endured. It was a not-so-gentle reminder of the seriousness of my surgery. Having felt so lucky throughout the process, I'd developed a tendency to minimize what I'd gone through. Dressing the wound and walking bent over by abdominal pain reminded me quickly, with no uncertainty, that transplant surgery had been a massive undertaking.

My fragility and the eruptions of pain made me a difficult patient. Audrey was ready. Her training and experience prepared her for patients like me. The more difficult things were for me, the more difficult things were for her. I knew she was worried. Not so much about my survival, but about seeing someone she loved suffering. I needed almost constant care at this point. Although I wanted to be a good patient, the pain exacerbated my vulnerability and created tension. The steroids made me emotionally labile—and every little thing that went awry became a possible point of contention. Seeing this new side of me, the kids were shocked and protective of Audrey; they didn't want her to bear the brunt of my volatility. She calmed their fears. Over time my mood stabilized and my reactionary outbursts declined. My steroid dose was also reduced, which helped to significantly decrease my irritability.

Two of Sarah's longtime friends, Molly O'Connor and Sarah Schwab, brought us dinner the evening of our first full day back home—the first of the many dinners prepared for us. Audrey's colleagues, the nurse anesthetists at NorthShore University HealthSystem, Evanston Hospital, signed up to cover the next two weeks of meals. Weave in our other friends' generosity, and we had a wonderful meal catered each night for the foreseeable future. The meals stabilized our lives and, most importantly, gave Audrey a breather from her long list of required tasks.

I tired quickly during the fun dinner provided by Sarah's friends that first night, and I went to bed early. Fortunately, I rested comfortably through the first night. Being home in my own bed was soothing. After an initial bout of pain from twisting and turning, I settled down. Sleep came soon, and the night passed uneventfully.

The next morning was calm and peaceful, and gratitude colored the start to my day. Everyone but me slept in. Rather than long, restful nights, my pattern was resting, dozing, and a few hours of real sleep. The lack of restful sleep was a problem that lingered for the next eight or nine months. The peacefulness of my first night at home was an exception.

Audrey caught me up on the CaringBridge posts from Saturday night while everyone else slept. Listening to the amazing comments people shared was a wonderful way to start the day and center me in my recovery.

On Sunday afternoon, Luke and I intended to watch the Bears game, which had long been a bonding experience for us. Terry decided to go to a bar to watch the Cleveland Browns game. Shockingly, Bret decided he'd go with Terry. We cautioned him, telling him it was too early and that rest was a far better option at this point. After all, he'd just had abdominal surgery to remove an organ. But Bret's determination convinced us to back off. Although he was part of the family, he wasn't our child. He was free to do as he wished. He returned six hours later in agony. Big mistake. Terry reported that Bret, even from his bar stool, helped prevent a bar fight. Bret's legend was growing by the day.

Luke made a CaringBridge entry:

> Sunday is the best time to sit back on the couch and watch some football, and that's exactly where we were. Bret was even able to make it to the bar earlier in the day to cheer on his hometown Browns. Along with watching the game, Bret could be seen keeping the peace when things got a little rowdy between some of the Cleveland and Oakland faithful. It seemed as though everything was back to normal as the fam ate some dinner later in the evening and watched a good ol' fashioned butt-kicking by Da Bears. Days like this will continue to remind the family of how lucky we are to have these two with us. Life is good.

I was resolute on walking that Sunday afternoon. My goal was one block, which seemed like a mile. Audrey and Emily came along. I was learning to walk all over again. Stooped over and creeping along, I made it around the corner and back. It felt like I was a hundred years old—feeble and weak. *What the hell happened? Had the surgery aged me forty years?* I still had a postsurgical shuffle. *God*, I thought, *I'm pathetic.* Despite my diminished capacity, walking became an everyday event. If I felt up to it, I did a short walk two or three times a day. Paradoxically, walking exposed my vulnerability but also provided a balance for it. As I got stronger, I added distance or time. In the days and weeks that followed, I waited for Audrey to come home. Other days a friend came over to walk with me. Leaving the safety of home brought unnerving trepidation, and having a caring friend along eased my anxiety. I felt so proud when I finished a walk, even the times when I needed to be propped up or caught if I stumbled. In those days of recovery, the walks replaced running for exercise. It was so gratifying to do something physical and normal. Consequently, my slow, affected ambling through the neighborhood became the benchmark for my healing and recovery. I had gone from being paralyzed by fear standing on a street corner, because I didn't know if I had the strength and speed to cross a traffic-less residential street, in the fall, to walking for an hour and a half before Christmas. When someone asked me how I was doing, my first response was to share the time or distance I roamed that day.

The repetition and frequency of my walks helped establish my recovery in those first days and weeks. The short hikes became a habit, but I tired easily and quickly so fatigue was almost always an issue. Taking the high dosages of steroids made sleep elusive. I dozed during the day sitting in my chair, but it wasn't restorative. At night, my sleep was fitful, and I dreaded needing to get up to use the bathroom. Pain accompanied any exaggerated movement. The ongoing, and supposedly normal, bleeding at the incision site scared me. I was struggling.

The highlight of my first weekend home was the time spent in the den when everyone was there. The mood was light and fun. I was ecstatic to have my family around me, and their company launched my recovery. From this starting point, my trajectory toward healing was established.

Having the CaringBridge entries read aloud to me—each morning and throughout the days—saw me through the times when I decompensated. The healing wishes strengthened all of us. We were flooded with blog entries on Sunday, October 16. There was an air of triumph and joy to them, as if my homecoming was being recognized as not only an accomplishment, but also a liberation from all that had transpired over the past eleven months.

Bret's sister, Lisa Jundi, wowed everyone with her entry:

> It was such a blessing to keep up with your updates. Although I've never met Greg or your family, you have been in my prayers steadily over the past couple of weeks. When I heard my brother was donating a kidney, I didn't even blink. I always said he would give his left arm for someone if he could, apparently I should amend it to the left kidney. My prayer was that both of you would come out well, and that the kidney would work well. I am so happy that the results have been so great, and from the reports my parents give, it couldn't have happened to a better person. I truly believe God worked a miracle and I am looking forward to meeting you some day. We will continue to keep you in our thoughts and prayers as you're recovering.

Lisa's comment about Bret's destiny confirmed my earlier speculation. It made us appreciate him even more.

The dedication of my family can't be overstated. Their presence, more than any of their considerable actions, was essential. I recognized how important it was for them to just be with me. The Andean shamans with whom I studied would say my family was "holding the space" in which I could recover. There's magic in the company of people who love you. I never felt alone. I was lifted up and humbled by the family's support and care.

Sunday evening Sarah called to tell her husband, Chris, that she was going to stay another couple of days. I remember her words: "I need to stay a few more days because I'm not feeling done yet." Being the loving, kind husband he is, Chris graciously supported her decision.

By Sunday evening, the family's rhythm was resetting to an acceptable "new" normal, one we all welcomed and felt safe in. The comfort of being home was transparent. Emily and Luke's earlier blog entries commented on how familiarity was apparent among us. The fading light of day washed over us and eased us into a calm, peaceful place. I sat in my chair and watched the Bears. Everyone was chatting and laughing. A sense of well-being permeated the house. *I made it*, I thought. It felt as if I was returning to a recognizable, normal state of being.

As Sunday faded into Monday, two tasks confronted us. The first was our appointment at the Transplant Clinic at eight o'clock Monday morning. It meant getting up at five o'clock and driving through downtown Chicago to Hyde Park. I dreaded the trip, but I knew it was crucial. *Why do I have to go back into the anxiety?* The second task was getting Bret checked out postoperatively and sending him back to Cleveland. Emily and Terry were staying long enough to drive him back.

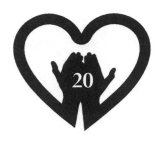

IT BEGINS—RECOVERY

On the occasion of every accident (event) that befalls you,
remember to turn to yourself and inquire what power you have
for turning it to use.

—Epictetus

Getting ready for my clinic visit Monday morning—waking up, showering, and leaving by five thirty—was hell. I doggedly stumbled, one foot in front of the other, through preparing for this necessary evil. En route to the hospital, Audrey, Sarah, and I saw a glorious sunrise on Lake Shore Drive; it was a good omen of what was to come. Other than suffering my self-induced fear of being driven, all went well. Propped up and handled gently by my family, we made it, intact, to the Transplant Clinic. Another milestone. My medical care was shifting from preparation and surgery to recovery, a clear sign I was making progress.

In the tension and confusion of us leaving the hospital the previous Friday, Bret's follow-up appointment had been scheduled for Wednesday, but Audrey had intervened and the appointment was moved to Monday to coincide with mine so he could get home sooner. After this first postsurgical visit to the clinic, Bret would bid us farewell and make the drive back to Cleveland with Emily and Terry. The plan was to wait until after our medical consults were completed to say our good-byes.

This visit included our first contact with Dr. Becker since the surgery. After my labs were done, we entered the exam room. Becker was waiting. Immediately, she went to work with her usual efficiency. I was shocked she wanted to remove the stitches, but out they came. She's a no-nonsense kind of doctor. My new kidney looked large and pronounced under the skin of my lower-right abdomen, about half the size of a football cut the long way. The size was, in part, due to postsurgical swelling. When Audrey asked if my "bump" would remain, Dr. Becker replied in the affirmative. I would have a permanent reminder—a protrusion from my lower-right abdomen—of my kidney transplant. No more six-pack abs or underwear modeling. I'd never been overly concerned with my physical appearance, but what vanity I had took a substantial hit with that revelation. Part of my healing, I began to understand, would be grieving the loss of how I'd looked before the surgery. My new reality meant, for example, that all my pants needed replacing. Welcome to elastic waistbands. In retrospect, I got the better end of the deal—a new life for the small price of vanity. But in moments of weakness, I still struggle to accept the resulting paunch.

And although I didn't realize it at the time, I wouldn't see Dr. Becker again. Timing and medical protocols would keep us apart. In retrospect, I also came to understand the practical nature of medicine. After playing her essential role in my survival, Becker moved on to help the next person in need of a transplant. That was her job, after all. The practice of medicine, like nature, is emotionless—cold, practical, and functional. Humans supply feelings and meaning to the miracles of medicine. The multitude of emotions I attached to her and what had transpired under her watch were my responsibility, and I learned to cope with them as I recovered and moved forward.

The major reason we chose UChicago for my transplant was the follow-up care they provide. Our decision was validated that morning. I knew going in that the medical staff was highly skilled, but I couldn't have anticipated their concern and compassion would match their professional excellence. It was love at first sight. The entire team was skillful, deliberate, and attentive. They didn't rush. I remember thinking that morning that this is how medicine should be practiced. Thorough doesn't adequately describe the attention to detail shown by Roseann, the nurse who treated me that morning. (How appropriate that she shared my sister's name.)

We learned the clinic protocol that visit: see the phlebotomist (blood draw), see nurse, see resident, see doctor, and then go home. Throughout the process, Sarah took notes, like the journalist she is. It was sweet to have her with us that morning and her thoughtfulness balanced a day that began with me grumbling. The focus of this first visit was to check the lab numbers to make sure the new kidney was working at an optimal level. Bret's kidney (and now mine) functioned flawlessly. My creatinine level was 1.1, and I was flabbergasted. Babies are born with creatinine like this. The flawless kidney was doing a "perfect" job. This news was the best possible and likely the most wonderful of my life. The reset button had been pushed—big time.

Roseann asked how I was feeling, meaning what percentage of normal I was experiencing in terms of what I could do. Initially, I said about 60 percent. As we talked and assessed my current condition, I realized it was actually about 30 percent. Although the pain was manageable, my activities and abilities were very, very limited. When I described how I struggled getting out of bed and the pain involved, it was evident a tremendous amount of my ability to function and care for myself was lost. I was impaired physically and diminished mentally. And to say my moods were unstable was an understatement. Life had changed dramatically. I needed to recognize and accept my reduced abilities and capacities—for the moment.

Because of the confusion regarding my medications when we left the hospital and our failure to bring the bottles of pills along to the appointment, Roseann insisted we come back on Wednesday to double-check the prescriptions. We didn't want to return so soon (especially me), but it was the best choice. It was an important post-op lesson: trust the process.

Audrey and Sarah were also impressed by the care at the clinic. It was a good day, but a long one. I would never have a short clinic visit, even though I was probably the healthiest transplant patient there. We were struck by how sick some of the other patients looked and how precarious their health seemed. My good fortune was clear: I hadn't felt "sick," even though I'd had end-stage renal disease, and I wasn't on dialysis prior to the transplant surgery. Also in my favor was that I had PKD (not diabetes), and I had a living donor. The tone, pace, and standard of care was being set for the next year of my recovery at the Transplant Clinic. I felt overwhelmingly positive about the future at this first visit. It was a comfort to know that some of the most knowledgeable and empathic people in medicine were going to oversee my care and recovery.

Bret's post-op visit went swimmingly. No surprise there. He couldn't have been healthier, given his recent kidney donation. Our fear was that because he was such an extraordinary physical specimen, he'd do too much too soon, which would impede his recovery. I grew increasingly aware of how much I didn't want Bret to suffer for being my donor. Audrey felt the same. Without intending to be overbearing, we persistently reminded him of our concerns. He agreed, told us what we wanted to hear, and then did what he was going to do anyway.

We later discovered Bret didn't take it easy those first few months. When we finally saw him again in April, there was concern he might have an incisional hernia from lifting too much. Emily, who remained in touch with Bret during those early months of recovery, reminded us that we couldn't protect or control Bret. How he approached living was the main reason he gave me the kidney. His lifestyle wasn't going to change because of the transplant or because he liked us.

Fittingly, our farewell to Bret at the Transplant Clinic included lots of tears. The bond of the relationship—forged through the intensity of the surgery, the drama we shared, and the magnitude of what Bret had done for me and the family—was powerful as we hugged, cried, and laughed in turn. Bret, the twenty-seven-year-old hero, stood among us, and our appreciation for his lifesaving gift flowed around and through us. Our gratitude will last a lifetime.

It was time for him to go. He was clearly ready, but I'm not sure I was. Although his kidney now resided in me, as long as he was present, an intense connection remained between him and it. His departure meant my new kidney and I would have to fly solo. After all the farewells were said and hugs given, he left. *I will hold you in my heart forever*, I thought as he walked down the hall flanked by Emily and Terry. It was fitting that Emily, who brought him to us, now took him safely home. We heard he was so exhausted, even though he refused to show it, the he slept the entire five-hour drive to Cleveland.

When we left the clinic, it was early afternoon, and I was utterly exhausted. This amount of activity, despite my sterling post-op report, far exceeded anything I had done for months. Upon our return home, I ate and then fell asleep in my chair. Rest was going to be essential. Getting healthier would evolve at its own pace, not at the rate I would choose. Additionally, being patient and making the requisite mental and emotional adjustments were crucial. My head and heart had to heal as much as my body did.

Audrey and I looked forward to the commotion surrounding the surgery dissipating. She planned to take a week off to keep a watchful eye on me. Her presence was incredibly comforting. I was embracing the idea of surrender, so I willingly turned my health over to her. The burden of my early recuperation fell squarely on her shoulders. Audrey was certainly more than capable, but the effort necessary came with a price. But at the moment, life after the transplant appeared manageable.

Sarah left Tuesday night to return to Chris and her job in Washington, DC. When everyone returned to where they belonged, the reality of what had transpired over the last six days (and eleven months) grabbed us. As the transplant stage of my adventure ended—as a smashing success—recovery began. Standing at the starting line to this final stage, the prospect of recovery was simultaneously exciting and daunting. It was a relief to be alone together for the first time in what felt like a long while. We faced the future with mixed feelings, though we were largely optimistic. Our magnificent start boded well for my future healing and recovery. But the acute risk of rejection was ever-present in that first month.

Audrey's presence calmed the troubled waters of my mind. I needed her now more than ever. As we settled into the "new normal," as she called it, all felt doable and peaceful. So far, so good.

THE NEW NORMAL

Experience is not what happens to a man; it is what a man does with what happens to him.

—ALDOUS HUXLEY

Wednesday—the one-week anniversary of the transplant—started with my second visit to the Transplant Clinic. It felt like I was in the movie *Groundhog Day*. The peace of Tuesday was gone, and I was back to the "work" of healing. We departed with little difficulty. The issue, which was a problem of my own creation, happened in transit.

Nervous about the journey, I harassed Audrey about her driving. She should have dropped me off on the side of Lake Shore Drive, gone home, and changed the locks. I was a jerk. I projected my fear onto her, and then felt guilty for it. Recognizing that's what I was doing was no excuse. Not my best moment. Maybe my worst. Fortunately, the tension I created dissipated when we arrived at the clinic. We had work to do. Audrey easily (it appeared) let go of my being an ass and treating her so poorly. In those days of recovery my shadow side reared its ugly head more than I like to admit. We acknowledged to each other that it was part of recovery, but I regret it and am embarrassed by it.

The clinic was consistent and the routine was the same—blood draw for labs, wait, check weight and vitals, go to an exam room, wait, be screened by the nurse, be seen by the resident, wait some more, and close with the nephrologist, who would prescribe meds. The second visit revealed my condition had changed. My liver enzymes were elevated. An ultrasound was scheduled for the next Monday. At the end of our visit, Dr. Patrick Cunningham assured us that we didn't need to worry. "We'll let you know when you need to worry," we were told, "and this is not the time." Their message calmed our shared fear. *Thank god. We dodged a bullet.* My other labs were stable—and, most importantly, my creatinine was 1.0. Thanks to Nurse Roseann's diligence, the medications were corrected. The steroid dose was reduced, and Ambien was prescribed to help me sleep. We cut our clinic time down from six hours on the first visit to four hours for this second visit.

Mostly because Audrey was a nurse anesthetist, we didn't have to return until Monday for the ultrasound. My labs needed to happen every other day, but they could be done at Evanston Hospital, just two miles from home. Substantial progress was made that morning. The clinic staff continued to impress. I was reassured that I was in good hands and that my treatment was superb. On the drive home, relieved and not overly concerned about liver enzymes (which reset to normal over the next week), my thoughts shifted to another task—making a blog entry. Humility and appreciation replaced my morning irritability.

After our clinic visit and almost one week after transplant surgery, I was determined to make an entry on the CaringBridge website. I was so moved and intrigued by what people were writing, including my own family members, that I wanted to say something to everyone who had become involved in my recovery and healing. With my medications keeping my sleep very light, the urge to write urgently surfaced in the middle of the night. The prednisone made me feel like I was sleeping in a clothes dryer. I was actively dreaming throughout the early hours of the morning, going in and out of an emotion-filled semiconsciousness.

A few nights earlier, I found myself dreamily composing a blog entry in my head. I was crying, then sobbing. Surprisingly, I didn't wake Audrey. Regardless of how the steroids affected me, it was a necessary catharsis. Rising early the next morning, I scribbled down everything I could remember of the blog post I'd written in my dream. As I did so, my thoughts took on an ethereal quality. It was difficult to distinguish between ideas from my conscious mind and unconscious thoughts. Those notes were the start of my first entry on CaringBridge, posted the afternoon of Wednesday, October 19:

> I think it's time I weigh in.
>
> Please remember that I'm still in that postsurgical state of mind and bear with me.
>
> It feels like eight days ago that Greg Baldauf went into the UChicago hospital and George Bailey of Bedford Falls came out. Instead of Zuzu's petals in my pocket, I've got Bret's kidney in my abdomen. This past week has been a lot like *It's a Wonderful Life*. You're all playing the part of Clarence.
>
> First and foremost, your words, your kindness, and your compassion have been inspiring for me and my family. Thank you for being witnesses to my journey and participating in it with your comments.
>
> The reading of your remarks usually starts early in the morning and continues until bedtime. This has become one of our fundamental rituals. Audrey or one of the kids read. I cry. Tears roll down my substantial cheeks and I have never felt more alive. More validated. More present. What a gift this has been for me. For us.
>
> I would almost recommend a kidney transplant . . . NOT!
>
> I want to talk about my immediate family: Audrey, Sarah, Emily, and Luke. I'll preface it by saying that I

think every parent wants to know how their children turn out. Well, I've gotten to find out. Sarah, Emily, and Luke showed up. They came through. Unsolicited. Unforced. They walked through this with me every step of the way. They were present throughout. They were brave and true. The sweet smiles on their faces, something I thought was lost to childhood, radiated the entire time. There is a fundamental goodness about them that is so powerful and healing that has touched me to the marrow.

Audrey, although you might prefer to be a rock star, you've been a rock. You haven't hesitated or wavered. You orchestrated this whole process from pillar to post. Or, as you would say, from tee to green. You have shown me the meaning of love, compassion, and commitment. Of all the blessings I've received, yours is the greatest. It's not difficult to see where the kids get their goodness from. Words don't do justice to what you have done and continue to do—so I'll simply say, from the heart, thank you.

Bret, my hero, I think we all want and need heroes. If you've ever been down and out, fearful or vulnerable, you have probably fantasized about someone swooping down and saving you. Bret did this for me. Incredible. The words of Tennessee Williams have new meaning to me: "I have always depended on the kindness of strangers."

All my life, from early boyhood, I've thoughts about heroes and courage. Perhaps this is the result of too many good-guy/bad-guy movies growing up. You know, questions like: "Would I go into the burning building to save someone?" "Would I jump in the river to save the drowning child?" "Would I fall on the grenade?" I think a lot of men think about things like this, but that's for another time.

Along comes Bret, a stranger. And do you know what he does? He jumps into the river. Only the river is me, and I get my life back. Wow. Hard to even fathom. Bret is very quiet. The strong, silent type. I may never really know why he did this. The best explanation I've gotten from him is, "It's the right thing to do." I'm left to think this is just who he is. I was very heartened by his sister's words a few days ago. Altruism is a part of his character, his personality, perhaps even his DNA. How cool is that? I envy his simple, elegant moral clarity.

Can you believe I'm the beneficiary of this miracle of strength and courage? Bret did this without flinching. He was steely-eyed, and he never veered from the course he set. His last words to me were that it wasn't that big of a deal. And he meant it.

Maybe we've all benefited. This is an amazing story. Life. Death. Courage. Real-life action. And, of course, a hero. The comments about Bret in the blog have been magnificent. He deserves as much praise as possible. I'm not sure he'll read them, despite my urgings. He's truly that modest and humble. They're worth saying anyway.

Life is richer and fuller for me right now. There is goodness and grace. I hope this is true for all of us. This moment of truth and beauty has left me feeling wonder and humility.

Thank you, Bret, for giving me my life back.

How about that for lofty thoughts? Let me bring it down to earth a little. Or "after the ecstasy, the laundry," to allude to one of Buddhist author Jack Kornfield's titles.

What a ride this has been. An absolutely wondrous convergence of forces made the hospital part of this go splendidly. Bret's exquisite kidney. My pristine vasculature. A world-class surgeon who got it done in two and a half hours. Home in three days.

My kidney function is now in the normal range. Am I lucky or what?

But there is another reality to all of this. My day-to-day life is about white-blood-cell counts, phosphorous levels, steroids and other pills, trips to the Transplant Clinic, and little sleep. I occasionally get shooting pains at the incision site. Normal, but it's no fun doubling over or grimacing. Deep, restorative sleep eludes me.

Audrey spends hours sorting pills. Pills, pills, and more pills . . . . Ugh. I peed twenty-six times on Monday. Is there a contest I can enter? When I ask what I could win, one of my family says "a healthy kidney." I've lost thirteen pounds of water weight since the beginning of the week. I discovered I have "pristine vasculature" but "weak abdominal walls." How's that for the balance of the universe? I'm literally learning to walk upright again. I've still got the postsurgical stoop going. My goal today is to walk two blocks.

It's going to be a long, challenging, and arduous recovery process. Slow and sometimes painful. There will be some bad days ahead. After a great Tuesday, I think I might have plateaued for a while.

But what a gift I've been given. I'll be learning to steward this gift. As I travel through all of this, I don't want to lose sight of that gift. I want to pay it forward as Sharon, my cousin and fellow transplant patient, has commented.

Thank you all for holding me in your hearts.

It is a wonderful life.

With love and gratitude,

Greg

The purge worked; I felt cleansed and restored after expressing the simultaneous emotions flowing just below the surface: relief, exhilaration, gratitude, exhaustion, vulnerability, anxiety, fear, and optimism. What a strange and exciting time it was. The intensity of our circumstance was rare and noteworthy, but we were too immersed in surviving to fully appreciate how amazing things truly were.

Life was changing rapidly. Today was merely the next step for us. Fortunately, Audrey was with me to guide me through the confusing malaise, answering my many questions and facing the myriad of challenges with me. She was an invaluable partner and friend. We recommitted to our early vow to be proactive.

When a person survives this type of down-and-dirty, intense, life-threatening situation, it's accompanied by a penetratingly real, rich, and rare opportunity. In those moments, I was living life to its fullest. Even the fear and anxiety I felt couldn't dampen the utterly incredible experience of being complete in the moment. I was living on the edge of the sword—we all were, in a way. The trick was to open my heart to it, commit to being fully present to enhance its impact and power. Initially, I was forced into this state of moment-to-moment presence by renal failure and the resulting transplant surgery. As time passed, I evolved; my consciousness elevated. My vulnerability was providing an opportunity to be better and courageous. I became more and more aware of what was happening. I wanted to cultivate and nurture this rare experience.

Sitting there that day, I was increasingly mindful of the critical roles played by awe and gratitude in this "peak" experience I was having. I was totally absorbed in these feelings. One week after the transplant surgery I thought, *Maybe I need to fasten my seat belt even tighter on this wild ride.*

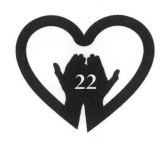

TRANSITIONS

Life must be lived as play.

—PLATO

I turned sixty on October 31, 2011. I was a Halloween baby. I relished the distinction of being born on such an interesting holiday; it shaped my personality. "Are you a trick or a treat?" I was asked growing up. Now, seventeen days after kidney transplant surgery, I again had fun with it. Here's my CaringBridge entry from October 30:

> Happy Halloween, everybody.
>
> I need your help. Because I'm essentially homebound and my activities are quite restricted (Audrey says I'm like a pet who can take walks and go to the vet), I need to be able to celebrate Halloween vicariously. As you may or may not know, Halloween is the greatest day of the year. Some of you may have mistakenly thought Christmas, New Year's Eve, or even your own birthday was. But I ask you, on what other day do strangers open their doors and give you treats? Plus, people wear costumes. See my point?

So if you're willing, I'm going to enlist you into the Great Pumpkin Army. The mission, if you choose to accept it, is to do as many of the following with a chortle, a chuckle, or chagrin.

Rock your bad self, or at least be a little naughty. (Please share the details.)

Befriend a little monster. Right, Lady Gaga?

Be the pumpkin . . . or at least carve one.

Spike the apple cider . . . or have a pumpkin latte.

Scare or be scared.

Boo it up.

Go trick-or-treating . . . or take someone.

Have the large size of a Snickers bar.

Trick it up tomorrow . . . or at least treat yourself well.

Take a ghost, goblin, or zombie to Starbucks.

If you pass a pumpkin patch, say hello to my peeps.

Ichabod your crane, but don't lose your head.

(My friend, John Tosto, reminded me the other day that having a captive audience like this may be a little dangerous for me.)

Here are a few things to keep in mind for tomorrow:

You're most likely to see a ghost during hypnagogia (the transition between sleep and waking).

One billion pounds of pumpkins are grown for Halloween. The state that produces the most? You guessed it—Illinois. Could this be in my honor?

Retailers make $600 million on this holiday.

The original treats were called *soul cakes*.

Please stay out of Grover's Mill, New Jersey, tonight. Orson Welles says the War of the Worlds will start there this evening.

Anyway, pay no mind to any of this. I'm on steroids.

Finally, I continue to do pretty well. The only thing missing is stamina. I've walked for over sixty minutes three days in a row. Unless Audrey's home, it's the highlight of my day.

Patty and Alan are coming over for chicken lamby pie tonight. I'll spend most of the morning at the Post-Transplant Clinic tomorrow. And Luke will come over for dinner tomorrow night. I got a flat-screen TV from the family for my birthday. Way cool.

All power to the Great Pumpkin.

Love you all,

Greg

Sarah responded:

DAD!

Happiest of sixtieth birthdays to you, Pops!

Soooo . . . did you get everything you were wishing for? ☺

So much love to you. Thank you, Mom, family, friends, and, of course, Super Bret, for making this October a life-altering experience. I'm feeling extremely lucky to have been a part.

Love to all on CaringBridge, especially you, Dad.

Turning sixty and transplant surgery were sobering life events. I was crossing a threshold—exiting my youth, a time when life lies ahead—and moving into my senior years, a stage of life that brings limits. I couldn't help but think I had more yesterdays than tomorrows. A lot could be said about turning sixty in a culture that overwhelmingly emphasizes being young or at least youthful. A line of demarcation clearly exists; aging and retirement merely confirmed it.

I'm not obsessed about aging or even particularly worried about it; I just accept it as an inevitable fact (to do otherwise is folly). But given the tenuousness of my situation, becoming sixty took on new meaning. I approached this birthday as if one life was ending and another was beginning. I didn't want to romanticize this milestone, but I knew I was at a crossroads. I had lived one life moderately successfully but fraught with mistakes and regrets; and now for reasons not completely clear to me yet, I was getting another one.

The Andean *paqos* (shamans) teach the importance of being *available* to life and experiences. You have to show up with an open heart and mind to whatever experience is at hand. If the potential exists for something amazing to happen, you first have to be present to experience it. That's when you discover things you can't learn in a book or by hearing about someone else's experience. Making myself available during my healing allowed me to fully engage what was happening. I believed I was living a miracle (a convergence of forces and events that resulted in amazingly positive outcomes). Many would choose to define this as a *sacred* event. I do.

That my kidney transplant occurred nineteen days shy of turning sixty steered me toward seeing the birthday as a harbinger of and the entry into the new life I would live after sixty. Perhaps turning sixty brought some wisdom with it. According to developmental psychologist Erik Erikson's psychosocial stages of development, sixty is when a person finds (or creates) meaning in the life they lived. I was right on schedule. I know the sixties are a generative time, and I was becoming acutely aware of the need to try to help others with PKD. Discussing that intention with Audrey cemented my desire to tell my story.

On November 2, I made this "Three Weeks after Surgery" entry on the CaringBridge blog:

> Hello, everybody,
>   First of all, thank you for all your birthday and Halloween wishes. It was a lot of fun hearing from you. You're all so gracious to indulge my pumpkin fantasies and play along.

It's amazing that I'm at the three-week mark. Wow. It's wonderful to be looking forward. Recovery and healing are far better than the stress of waiting. What a month October was. I hope I never have another quite like it.

I believe I can unequivocally say I'm doing quite well overall. With a few exceptions, each day usually brings some improvement. This process has been incredible. I never imagined this would go so well and I would be so fortunate. I realize I'm not out of the woods yet. The acute rejection phase lasts for months, but the volatility decreases with each passing day, week, and month.

So as the drama and intensity wanes, I'm left with the mundane, day-to-day process of healing. Ultimately, it's a long, slow process. Although I feel somewhere from OK to good, the clinic folks tell me I'll start feeling great at around six weeks. Can't wait.

The very good news is that my creatinine is 1.3, which is in the normal range. I have normal kidney function. *Holy shit!* It's been thirty-five or forty years since that's been true. I also found out Monday that my HDL cholesterol is 63. I haven't seen that number since I ran the marathon in '88.

The minor annoyances are sleep, steroids, and stamina with some incision pain thrown in for good measure. The first two are related. The steroids have an adverse effect on my sleep. Lately they wake me up at around 4:30 in the morning. I stay in bed until 5:00, but I never feel very rested. The good news is that they've begun to reduce my steroid dosage and, hopefully, this will resolve itself. In the future.

Stamina is what I don't have. I can select activities. I got up to walking for an hour, but afterwards, I'm done and in the chair. Because of some bleeding at the incision site, they've suggested

I dial back my walking for a week. I'm glad I don't have to do anything important.

All of this is relatively minor, and I'm blessed to be where I am now.

I can't make a journal entry without acknowledging all the support my family and I have received. It has made a huge difference in my recovery. The words, cards, meals, and love have been tremendous. My life has been forever changed for having this experience.

I ran across something in a book I've been reading—*The Spirituality of Imperfection* by Ernest Kurtz and Katherine Ketcham, which I highly recommend—that has helped me understand what's been happening. Briefly, it's a little model of growth that has four phases: surrender (what could be more of a surrender than surgery?); gratitude for the gift that has been given; humility and giving up control; and tolerance (acceptance). I'm finding that this describes the process of what I've been going through. Works for me.

Be well. More next week.

With love and gratitude, Greg

My recovery kept progressing through early November. I was writing more on the CaringBridge blog. Popular demand kept it afloat. Because we'd developed something of a following, I felt obliged to keep people informed. I wrote the following on November 9:

Hello, everybody!

Well, today marks four weeks from my transplant surgery. Incredible!

In some ways the time has flown by; in other ways, it has crept or plodded along. But without a doubt, I'm glad to be where I am today. Four weeks of healing and four weeks into a new life.

To cut to the chase, according to the nurse at the Transplant Clinic, after reading my lab results yesterday, the kidney is working "perfectly." This really tells the whole story; everything else is minor in comparison. My amazingly good fortune continues. I will add that I'm quite sure that's the only perfect thing about me. I'll take it, though, and smile. Thank you, Bret. Your gift keeps on giving and I remain humbled by its magnitude.

The day-to-day stuff moves slowly. With Audrey back to work, it's very quiet here, especially around three to four in the afternoon. I appreciate the calls and the visits. They're wonderful distractions. People have been so damn wonderful to me. I sometimes ask myself if they have the right person.

Audrey added a medical update on November 12:

All is well with the kidney, that's the big thing. We said we knew things wouldn't always be smooth, but it does disarm us when the bumps happen. Not a great couple of days for my guy. Yesterday he had a bit of a scare with the incision bleeding, after four weeks—really?—not fair. That seems to be under control, but the other thing that has been nagging him is a reaction to the meds (mostly the steroids, we think), feeling shaky and a bit out of it. Today it has lasted most of the day, though usually it's pretty short-lived. Just a little reminder that this is *not* for sissies. He's not a complainer and would probably not want me writing this, but I think a realistic view of what he's dealing with is what people who care about him want. I'm hoping tomorrow will be a better day. I hope the Bears give him a win.

Thanksgiving was fast approaching. With family and friends gathering, we were about to celebrate my second-favorite holiday. I had some work to do. Until this point, I'd had no desire to get behind the wheel; it petrified me. My reflexes and coordination were out of whack. I thought I could kill someone. Practice was the only way to quell my fear.

One sunny afternoon in mid-November, I got in the car, backed out of the driveway, and drove to Lake Michigan, about two and a half miles away. I desperately wanted to confront and overcome my vulnerability. Slowly, cautiously, and gripping the steering wheel with all my might, I made it without incident. I sat in the parking lot and stared at the lake. It was gorgeous. The reward for facing my fear was beauty. Drinking in how lovely the world looked in those moments was a celebration of my small but significant accomplishment. My meditation and celebration abruptly ended with one thought: *I have to drive home. Ugh!* Slightly tense, my vulnerability manageable, a bit more confident, with a lighter grip on the wheel, I proceeded home. *Victory!*

On the Sunday before Turkey Day, Audrey wrote another CaringBridge post:

> I had hoped Greg would be doing the update, but he's not quite up to it. Our clinic visit on Wednesday elicited many glowing reports about what Bret's/ Greg's kidney is doing. They're truly amazed. I don't think this is a common outcome, so we're very blessed and thrilled about that. Steroids have been lowered to the dose he will remain on forever (according to UChicago protocol), so sleep has been *much* better. All of that is fabulous news, but he's still getting his butt kicked by a side effect of one of the anti-immune drugs, he feels jittery, shaky, and kind of out of it. Some days are better than others, but it's with him most days. Kind of getting him down a bit. He was told he'd feel *great* by six weeks, which is Wednesday. We have a ways to go for that.

Thanksgiving has a simple elegance to it, which I love. I adore its singular theme—gratitude. Family and friends gather, you eat and watch football on TV. Maybe a board game gets thrown in to round out the festivities. This year, the meaning of the day was amplified. I wrote this on CaringBridge the day before Thanksgiving 2011:

> Happy Thanksgiving, everyone!
>
> Today marks the sixth week from my transplant surgery. Hard to believe, but it's true. Time is relentless; but in this case, it's a gift.
>
> I'm feeling pretty damn good the last three days. This is the longest run I've had. I've even driven the last two days (just to the lake and the hospital). More importantly, as of last Wednesday, my lab numbers continue to be "perfect." Hallelujah! This is cause for great joy and optimism. Bret's kidney is working like a champ, and I thank God, the Great Spirit, and the heavens above for this. Having the kidney work so beautifully puts everything in perspective. I'm truly a lucky man.
>
> Last Wednesday, the stent (a routine part of the transplant surgery to keep the ureter, a passageway between the kidney and bladder, open so fluid can flow through it) was removed. Mercifully, it happened quickly—less than sixty seconds. They don't even give you a bullet to bite on. I survived . . . with minimal discomfort.
>
> More good news: my creatinine is 1.4 as of today, which is nothing short of amazing. The steroids have been reduced to five milligrams, which is the maintenance level I'll be on for a long while. And I'm sleeping seven to eight hours a night. Being able to sleep is such a relief and helps so much. It makes the return to normal possible.
>
> My current struggle—one seems to follow the other—has been a reaction to the medication, specifically Prograf (tacrolimus), which is one of the antirejection medicines. Essentially, after my morning dose, my hands shake. If it intensifies,

which it has a couple of times, I feel drugged or in a stupor. But when it's bad, it's like being hit in the head with a baseball bat. I think adjusting to the meds is going to be one of the bigger challenges I'll face. I can't imagine functioning at any significant level feeling like this. We'll see what happens.

I'm waiting for my lab results this afternoon.

The kids sent me a T-shirt with the best reframing of having a kidney transplant I can imagine: "I have 3 kidneys. KAPOW. What's your superpower?"

Bret is up near Chautauqua, New York, at deer-hunting camp. He shot an eight-point deer last weekend. From my point of view, he deserves to get whatever makes him happy. However, I haven't had the urge to buy a shotgun.

Thanksgiving is tomorrow, and the Baldauf family will be joyously assembling in Evanston over the next few days. I'm glad they're coming here, because it'll be much easier for me than having to go someplace else. The girls are promising to help Audrey cook.

I have a strong feeling that Thanksgiving will be extra special for me this year. The normal feelings of thanks and appreciation are certainly heightened. . . . I'm swimming in gratitude. When life has been given or extended in such a transparent fashion, it creates in me tremendous wonder, joy, and humility.

So at the Thanksgiving table tomorrow with my family, this awareness will be very present. I hope it lasts a long time. I don't want to lose the feelings or the new awareness.

Thank you for being a part of my healing journey and return to wholeness. You have given me a magnificent gift that I will cherish forever.

With love and gratitude, Greg

P.S. UChicago just called, and all three numbers remain excellent. Yay!

With so much to be thankful for, the timely significance of this holiday left me feeling extremely humble. The premeal ritual of going around the table and sharing what you're thankful for took on new significance. I made myself *available* to this experience. Sitting at that table, in that moment, was electric.

Buoyed by the exhilaration of Thanksgiving, I began to think of the future, at least the immediate future the new year would bring. Returning to work entered my mind for the first time. Because I was retiring in the summer of 2012, I wanted to finish my career by working my final semester. Teaching that last semester became a persistent goal, ever-present in my mind as my recovery moved consistently forward. But first I had to make it through Christmas and New Year's celebrations.

In order to stay on the trajectory of my recovery and encouraged by my earlier drive to the lake, I drove a little every day until I felt I could make the ten-mile trip to the college without hurting anyone. My first goal was to attend a staff meeting in early December. Although driving remained an issue for the next eight months, through practice, I diminished my anxiety enough to expand the number of normal activities I could accomplish. These initial ventures back to normalcy bridged my healing and recovery to the life I knew before the surgery. These two acts—driving and attending a staff meeting—launched me back into living as opposed to convalescing. They were crucial milestones.

I thought of the staff meeting as a rehearsal for returning to work for real in January. Attending it was a huge leap in my recovery. My choice to get "back on the horse" reflected a trust that my healing would continue for the foreseeable future. But still, I routinely struggled with opposing thoughts: the future was both exciting and intimidating. I wanted to get better, but not exceed my diminished capabilities. I worried that I was going too fast, too soon. These oppositions are the paradox at the heart of recovery. *How do I progress, but not fail by overdoing it?* My acute sense of vulnerability and anxiety were remedied by small accomplishments, despite the angst and worry that were ever-present. Mentally and emotionally this was how my recovery moved forward; these were the challenges I faced on a daily basis.

The plan was to miss the week in January before classes start, which is when faculty usually return to campus. That would allow an additional week of recuperation in Florida. With her customary grace and style, Joi, my administrator, told me to do whatever I needed to do to take care of myself. I was extremely fortunate to have the support and freedom to act in my own best interest during my recovery.

During this time my new kidney continued to perform magnificently. My blood work and clinic visits were excellent. My walking improved in distance and speed. I was up to about an hour every day, with less need to stop or rest. I asked the nurses and doctors when I could exercise. They cautioned me to wait. I did so willingly, but the request was an indicator of my continued healing. My progress was atypical for most transplant patients. About 20 percent of kidney transplant patients have a rejection episode and about 5 percent reject the kidney outright. Why was I so privileged to avoid those outcomes? Despite often feeling guilty about my good fortune, I eventually accepted the gift given me.

JUMPING THE SHARK

Everything has been figured out, except how to live.

—Jean-Paul Sartre

The Christmas season began in earnest. The holidays were another marker of my recovery. Spending time with people who care about me was stimulating and satisfying; and, with Audrey back at work, the anticipation and preparations interrupted the tedium of being alone.

December 12 was the two-month anniversary of my surgery. Most significantly, this landmark signaled the opportunity to exercise, which would validate my progress. Medical consent was given for a light workout a week later. Lifting the exercise ban turned out to be a blessing and a curse in the vein of the saying "Be careful what you pray for." I yearned for more strenuous physical activity beyond the walking I'd been doing, thinking it would demonstrate that I was *really* healing; but in hindsight I recognize that my enthusiasm had long-term consequences. I would've been better off tempering my overzealous estimation of the importance of exercising at that stage of recovery. But I so wanted to feel strong and not vulnerable. Unfortunately, my intentions—to gain strength and stamina and not be weak and helpless—didn't match the result. I went to the gym twice that week before Christmas. In the moment, I was excited and proud of my accomplishment. *If I can exercise*, I thought foolishly, *there's nothing I can't do.* Sadly, my efforts resulted in a large hernia a year later.

On Monday, December 12, at 4:02 p.m., I made this CaringBridge entry:

> Hello, everybody!
>
> Here I am two months past the transplant. Amazing.
>
> I thought I would give you an update about what's happening.
>
> All is well. In fact, it's better than that. At about the six- to seven-week mark, I started feeling quite a bit better. I noticed I was walking faster and generally felt like I had turned a corner. The things that were bothering me, like reactions to the meds, seemed to dissipate. I started thinking I might be ready for the next step.
>
> So I went back to Oakton for a meeting last week. Now before you think this is too soon—I'm not working regular hours. The folks who've been subbing for me in my classes are still in place. But I really wanted to return before the end of the semester to see my students, friends, and colleagues. Although it gets tiring, overall I've been energized by the return to a more normal life. This is an important goal for me to reach, and emotionally it's been very satisfying. Only my good buddy Cary has told me that he doesn't want to hear about my kidneys anymore. He even asked me how many minutes I spend talking about them. What are friends for?
>
> My lab results, the ultimate indicator of my recovery and overall health, continue to be "perfect." In fact, Audrey's comment last Wednesday upon seeing the numbers was, "This is the first time I can ever remember seeing labs for you that had no red

numbers." Everything was in the normal range. So when you're toasting this holiday season, celebrate this for me.

Among the many cool things that have happened in my life lately is that Emily volunteered to head the local PKD chapter in Cleveland. She recently spent a day in Kansas City at the headquarters of the National PKD Foundation getting inspired and finding out more about this disease. I'd say it's an excellent example of someone paying it forward. Em, you do us all proud! Very classy.

It's hard to believe I'm at this point. It was just a year ago on December 17, 2010, that I found out a transplant was headed my way. When I see that date again in a few days, I'll have almost ten weeks of recovery completed. Things happen fast.

Bret is doing well. There's a possibility he might be visiting us this weekend with his daughter, Hadley. His one condition for giving me the kidney was that we have a scotch together. I can finally have that drink with him now.

I have a lot to celebrate this Christmas and New Year. I'm very happy to be here, to be healing as well as I am, and to have the support and love of family and friends. Thanks again for all your kindnesses these past few months. It's been instrumental in my recovery.

Unless something unforeseen happens, my plan is to make one more journal entry at the three-month mark in mid-January. From what I've read, three months is an important milestone. The farther away from the surgical date, the stronger I'll get and the less risk I'll have for rejection. My immune system will get stronger, but it'll never be at the level it was before the transplant.

That's all I've got.
Have a great holiday season.

With love and gratitude, Greg

How quickly things can change. I awoke on December 23 intending to go back to the gym for a third time; instead I went to the ER. By midmorning, I was on the couch writhing in pain. Initially, I thought the anguish was a result of exercising. But because the painkillers I took were ineffective, I realized something far more serious might be occurring. The agony intensified and the situation became alarming, bringing the worst-case scenario to mind—rejecting the kidney. All along the threat of a rejection episode was always lurking, but it had receded because I felt so good. Still, nothing like a bout with severe abdominal pain to bring that fear charging to the fore.

By early afternoon, after telephoning the nurse on call at the Transplant Clinic, it was obvious I was headed to Evanston Hospital's emergency room. What a horrible start to the Christmas weekend. Sarah, who had arrived early to help with my care if need be, was dumbfounded by my sudden turn for the worse. Having heard the stories of my wonderful progress, she was seeing me at my lowest point since the transplant surgery. Echoing the nurse's recommendation, Sarah was resolute that I should go to the hospital immediately. Off we went.

Going to a hospital emergency room on a holiday weekend is awful. And even Audrey's long tenure at Evanston Hospital held no sway in an ER scenario. We waited in line just like everyone else. After the admission screening, then entry into the ER, the usual drill commenced. No pain medication would be given until the appropriate tests were done. We settled in for the long haul. An IV was started and my temperature taken. Curiously, as was my typical ER pattern, I began to feel better. The pain subsided—maybe due to a placebo effect because I believed treatment was at hand.

Fortunately, the ER doc willingly consulted with Dr. Nash, my regular nephrologist in the Evanston Hospital system, who recommended the most kidney-friendly antibiotics and painkillers. One of the few flaws at UChicago's Transplant Clinic was the lack of an on-call nephrologist. Nash's availability for a consult was a tremendous help. Preliminary tests were normal, but the deciding one, the CAT scan, required an additional wait. And true to ER form, so did the results. Fortunately, Audrey did have some influence in Interventional Radiology, where a CAT scan was done. Because she frequently administered anesthesia there during her workday, I got bumped up on the waiting list. However, nothing could change the time it took to get the results.

Finally, the ER doctor got the results from the radiologist. Apparently one or more of the cysts on my old kidneys ruptured. I'd experienced ruptured cysts a few years before, being in end-stage renal disease. My current situation was very similar. Why having a cyst burst now was so painful was unclear, but apparently PKD wasn't done with me, bringing me to my knees and to the ER. I went home exhausted and frustrated. This incident was the first major setback of my recovery. My early progress had allowed me to delude myself into thinking I had an unobstructed path to recovery and health. Surprise! I got a resounding wake-up call—a whack upside the kidney.

We usually celebrate Christmas Eve with Audrey's side of the family at her sister Maizie Grisch's home in Aurora, Illinois. We all assumed this long-standing tradition would continue. Sarah and Chris even made a special trip this year to participate. Even though I was tired and shaky from the previous day's trial, I intended to make the fifty-mile trip for some Christmas cheer.

As the morning progressed, it became transparent that my capacity to partake in the Christmas Eve celebration was in jeopardy. I anticipated Audrey's disappointment. Not seeing her family would be a setback for her. When I was certain I couldn't travel, I pleaded she go without me. Initially she agreed. But by midafternoon, my temperature went above one hundred degrees, a red alert for a transplant patient. A fever was potentially threatening and could lead to a rejection episode. The alarm went off. We contacted the on-call nurse, Mary Beth. (It's never good to be an on-call nurse on a holiday.) When she answered the phone, it was apparent that she was at her family's holiday celebration. I felt guilty for bothering her. She urged us to go back to the ER. Her most persuasive point: "Why risk losing a wonderful kidney because you didn't go to the ER?" What a way to convince us and make her point crystal clear. Off we went. Again.

Although moved to action by the clarity of Mary Beth's words, as we drove to the ER, our reticence was stirring. We really didn't want to visit the ER on Christmas Eve. We began to ask ourselves if my temperature was truly indicating an infection. Our fear of kidney rejection coupled with Mary Beth's urging overcame our reluctance. But when the ER nurse told us my temperature was normal, we broke rank. Fear was replaced by reason, anxiety by calm. Except for leaving the hospital after the transplant surgery despite conflicting dosage instructions for my medications, we'd always complied with medical advice. In this situation, we chose to act in our best interest based on the available information. To be sure we weren't being reckless, we waited an hour and had my temperature and blood pressure taken again—still normal. Our ER visit came to an abrupt halt. Our mission was aborted, and home we went.

What a miserable two days! Along with some cysts, my bubble had burst. As if the ER visits weren't enough, I also felt sluggish and weak. Reviewing what I had gone through, I realized how tenuous my recovery truly was and how fragile and frail my condition. What a reality check. Heeding the warning shot across my bow, my attitude shifted. I relinquished my claim of a rocket-like trajectory back to health. So ended that fantasy. These Christmas events showed me that I needed to reassess and adjust my strategy about recovery.

Christmas Day, even though I was subdued, was quite wonderful and temporarily lifted me out of my doldrums. Being with Audrey and the kids as well as my sister, Roseann, and her children was joyous. I couldn't have scripted a better holiday celebration. The festivities balanced the previous two days' turmoil. We noted the difference of this Christmas from the previous one, which had included our clumsy effort to share the horrible news about my renal failure. What a difference a year makes. The day ended with our family discussing that we truly might have touched the meaning of Christmas—joy and love. We all agreed this Christmas was a thousand times better than the year before.

One holiday task remained, the annual post-Christmas family dinner and theater outing. Audrey would buy tickets to the hottest production in town, and we'd go to our favorite Chicago steakhouse, Smith & Wollensky on State Street, where it intersects the Chicago River. We'd consume an extravagant steak dinner, gaze down "State Street, that great street" (immortalized in the Sinatra song), and enjoy a glorious night out on the town. This year we unanimously decided to pass on our tradition because of my risk of infection or getting sick. This adventure would've been my first time in a large crowd since the transplant. Up to this point, my limited excursions were walks to Starbucks, medical visits, and my visit to the college. Our plan was modified. As a compromise that would shorten the evening and reduce the moving parts, we went to the famous improv-comedy club in Chicago, Second City, and a restaurant next door to it. No one seemed to mind. The play and dinner left me exhausted, but I forced myself to participate. After such overwhelming support for months, I didn't want to disappoint or let everyone down. I controlled my anxiety to a manageable level and showed up. But afterward, I was drained, and I couldn't wait for the holidays to end. I craved inactivity and quiet. I wanted life to slow down again so that I could resume a softer, steadier pace of recovery.

A few days later, we found peace and quiet in Florida, where we'd long been planning to retire. At my last clinic visit, clearance was given to travel and, fortunately, not rescinded because of my yuletide ER visits. We left town, but in a much more vigilant frame of mind.

It was now ten weeks since my surgery, and this life-altering year was drawing to a close. Although still weak and tired from hitting the pothole of ruptured cysts, I was cautiously optimistic about going away. I was also disconcerted by the knowledge that my rest period was winding down—and my worries were growing about being sufficiently recovered to return to work in January. However uncertain, I remained committed to what I perceived as the next step in my recovery. Pushing the reality of returning to work from my mind, I focused on the warmth of sunny Florida and the promise of rest. Life would accelerate soon enough.

I woke up Thursday morning, December 28, feeling wobbly. My goal that morning was to get on a plane to Florida. Doubts persisted, but I believed the rest and relaxation would rejuvenate me. However, believing this didn't prevent feeling numb and slow. Audrey was concerned. My condition required her patience, a familiar attitude for her the past thirteen months. The cab arrived; we left for the airport. Our determination prevailed despite our misgivings.

At the airport, I cautiously navigated the crowded hallways and the security line. It was striking how vulnerable I felt in public. The airport seemed oppressive and crazy. *Don't think; keep moving*, I told myself. Arriving at the gate, we discovered our seats were changed because of modifications in the flight schedule. We were separated and seated in the rear of the plane. Audrey worked her magic to ensure we got the seats she'd reserved. She used a gambit we called "the kidney thing," telling the airline representative about my recent kidney transplant and that I needed to be cared for during travel (not untrue). Mistakenly (and amusingly), the airline official thought I was carrying a kidney for a transplant in Florida. I simply watched this unfold from afar, smiling and keeping my mouth shut. When the airline official approached us to ask if we needed to keep the kidney refrigerated on the plane, I almost burst out laughing. We sat in the first row.

On the plane, after watching that little drama occur, a familiar refrain returned: I was not in control, at all. I was caught up in the momentum of evolving circumstances—not only in the current context, but continuously. At that point, I did the smart thing; I let go, which allowed me to relax and change my attitude. The low energy I was currently experiencing was replaced by an energy that was more fluid and flexible. This shift I felt on that flight to Florida was the beginning of a larger change.

We arrived unscathed. The trip south, despite my early ruminations and hesitations, was ultimately uneventful. Boring and dull are the only way to travel. My friend Bernie met us at the airport and welcomed us back to the land of sun and palms. The gulf breezes felt comforting and invigorating. Just being out of the Chicago winter lifted our spirits. Bernie, who had been a loyal, caring friend throughout my ordeal, made us feel welcome. We returned to a community of Florida friends we'd been part of for ten years. Caring, concern, and compassionate relationships continued to loom large in my recovery.

Our home in Venice was eerily quiet when we entered, and the air was stuffy and stale. Opening the doors and windows that had been closed since the previous May brought energy and life back to it. The house breathed in the fresh air, and so did we. Our familiar and soothing Florida routine revived us. What a departure from visits to the ER and the hum of the holidays. As our pace slowed, we absorbed the tranquility. Our sole purpose was to relax. The numerous tasks, jobs, and goings-on associated with survival were left behind in Evanston.

Within a day, a curious thing happened. I started feeling better, but Audrey got sick. With each passing hour, I felt energized and Audrey felt worse, barely able to move off the couch. The strain of the past three months—not to mention the stress of the past year—had pushed Audrey past her limit. Forced to be strong and unwavering for so long, her body rebelled. With my relative stability, she let her guard down. She buckled, unable to muster enough energy to even have fun. Along with some flu- and cold-like symptoms, it was apparent she was exhausted. Her body cried out for rest. Fortunately, rest was all she had to do.

Meanwhile, with her permission and encouragement, I went about the business of being in Florida. I played a little golf and saw friends on a limited basis. My independent activities created a respite for her. She didn't have to take care of me. I even celebrated New Year's Eve with our Florida friends by myself for a few hours. She was deeply asleep by the time I returned home before ten o'clock. The new year began alone, but knowing Audrey was recovering in the next room gave me a deep sense of serenity and calm.

It was now 2012, and our optimism was renewed. I was shocked to feel so good. The setback of Christmas Eve and its residue retreated. Being physically active left me feeling tired, and my weariness was an important reality check. My pre-Christmas experiences had taught me to pay close attention. I could play golf or walk on the beach, but there were limits. If I exceeded them, I felt depleted. During the three weeks we stayed in Florida, I tested those boundaries. I learned a lot about my capacity for activity, discovering I was able to do *one* activity per day but rarely a second.

I had one "awful, terrible, very bad day" that forced me to the couch. I recovered quickly—another lesson learned. My body reset naturally. Physical recovery—in a short amount of time—was something I hadn't experienced for quite a while. Never dreaming I could play golf three months after the operation, I shot an 83, close to my lowest round ever. Audrey also recovered, but it took a week before she'd bounced back sufficiently for her favorite Florida activity—walking on the beach.

As my strength and stamina stabilized, I mentally started preparing to return to teaching. It loomed large on the horizon, growing in significance as the date neared. I wanted to finish my thirty-four-year career with momentum and grace, rather than stumble to an ignominious end, but I had lingering reservations about my ability to do so. Oddly enough, the seemingly frivolous act of golfing helped me assess my physical capacity to get back to work. Although I was active for a transplant patient, I relied on the luxury of being able to sit or lie down at any time to recuperate. Back at work, I wouldn't be able to structure my day around resting whenever I got tired. My days on the golf course built my confidence about sustaining my energy when I was back at work.

When we left Florida, I felt stronger and slightly optimistic. *Bring it on,* I thought. I returned home as ready, able, and willing as possible to teach my classes in two days.

STRUGGLING, BALANCING,
SUCCEEDING

Life is a tragedy when seen in close-up,
but a comedy in long-shot.

—CHARLIE CHAPLIN

My return to Oakton Community College was fantastic. I was welcomed with open arms. My colleagues and Joi, the vice president of student affairs, were reassuringly supportive, gracious, and helpful. After the first day, I knew all the ingredients were present to make my transition back a success. All I had to do now was stay healthy.

The kind welcome of my colleagues was heartening. People stopped me in the hall or poked their heads in my open office door to ask how I was doing. I found myself tearing up after someone dropped by my office or gave me a hug. Their random acts of kindness reinforced my recovery and healing, though I doubt my colleagues realized the effect they were having. My heart and soul were being fed, restored, and filled in new ways.

As the life-changing events were unfolding over recent months, I was making discoveries that profoundly shifted my perceptions.

Although my recent life was completely absorbed by a life-threatening disease, illness, surgery, and recovery, I was also playing a part in a broader existential, or perhaps spiritual, drama. Just living and confronting challenges as they arose from day to day had forced me to take dramatic action, which compelled me to redefine what began as a physical crisis into an evolving emotional and spiritual experience.

I began to realize how this phenomenal series of events falls into a precept I learned from the Andean paqos—"It cannot be taught; it can only be experienced." Being lifted by love and compassion was healing in the most expansive sense—for the mind, body, heart, and soul. It reached the core of my being. I let these healing moments, these daily miracles, wash over me at every opportunity. They sustained me when I struggled or stumbled, helping move me forward. I was slowly becoming whole again—the definition of healing.

A deep, deep sense of gratitude and wonder at the sheer *goodness* of people continued to emerge. Life and living were affirmed. I'd experienced love in my life before. After all, my immediate family and close friends were spectacular in caring for me and watching over me during my most difficult times. But I can readily say I'd never experienced love in this magnitude before. The incantation used to open sacred spaces for shamanic rituals includes the wonderful phrase: "Open my heart so that I can see." As my heart expanded, my vision shifted, and I realized I was experiencing the world differently. How ironic that a life-threatening disease and its resulting vulnerability led to such an astonishing awareness about the human condition: as much as people need to be loved and nurtured, they also need to love and nurture. What I had once only known intellectually was now revealed through the literal events of my life, which made them more tangible and real.

An additional insight emerged at this time in my recovery. People love you in the ways available to them. Often they love you as they would like to be loved. A person's capacity to love differently is based on their life experiences, histories, and belief systems. People express love and care the best they're able. Some people love grandly and easily and are capable of great generosity. Others are more restricted and limited in their ability to give, parceling out their love with precise measure. The ways people love are as varied as the people themselves. But we all love. With this awareness in mind, I was able to take love into my heart and allow it to help heal me. Being the beneficiary of love also facilitates a person's ability to love. As I read *The Spirituality of Imperfection* by Kurtz and Ketcham I resonated with the idea that being loved and being forgiven allow a person to love and forgive. I was empowered to love the people around me. Recognizing this dynamic was yet another gift to me.

My first two classes of my last semester of teaching were scheduled for my second day back. I was flat-out scared. I hadn't been in front of a group of people in three months. Although I loved teaching and thought I was reasonably competent, it felt like I was walking into the classroom for the first time. Feeling fatigued as I sat at in my office the hour before my class, I thought, *Bad sign if I'm this tired before I even start.* Much to my surprise, though, walking into the classroom energized me. It was as if I were catapulted forward into performance mode and simultaneously backward into the familiar comfort of what I'd been doing for more than thirty years. I pulled it off and got through that class and the next with little or no damage done to my students or myself.

After I finished classes that first day and stumbled back to my office, I collapsed into my chair, totally spent. I'd survived. Although there was a long way to go—sixteen weeks—I didn't crash and burn on my first teaching attempt after the transplant. As I slowly recuperated, I mentally and physically prepared myself for the drive home. When I arrived, I curled up on the couch. As my strength returned, a very satisfying feeling washed over me the rest of the afternoon and evening. Enduring this day was a small triumph.

Completing that first week set the tone and pattern for my last semester as a college professor. Initially it required a significant effort to get started every morning. I hadn't had a daily schedule of any kind for over three months. Gradually, an acceptable routine was established; and over time, I was able to put in a full day. But I discovered work was all I could do. When I got home in the late afternoon, I was finished for the rest of the night. It was a continuation of what I'd learned in Florida—one activity per day was fine, but two couldn't be sustained.

My abundant limitations left me fairly useless when it came to participating in the routine running of a household. Consequently, Audrey was forced to take over the mundane, domestic chores. Her responsibilities seemed endless then and overwhelming in retrospect. She was all goodness, grace, and style—and she met the challenges without protest. She also cheerfully put up with my mood shifts and grumpiness. But as the days and weeks passed, it was apparent that she was beginning to tire. The massive extra effort I required on top of her demanding job took a toll. She slept more and showed signs of being sick: upset stomach, increased aches and pains, feeling run-down.

My daily travails were replaced with some truly magnificent news. Sarah officially announced she was pregnant. Life changed lanes again for me and us. The energy of survival surrounding the family for over a year was transformed into the energy of renewal and new life. The brightness of Sarah's declaration replaced the angst of returning to teaching and the focus on the daily struggles we encountered. Audrey's burden was replaced by anticipation and joy. Having already received many gifts, the impending birth of our first grandchild, was the ultimate one.

My teaching settled into a reasonable and comfortable pace. As long as I stayed within my limits by not overdoing things or taking on too much, I performed like my old self (or at least a reasonable facsimile). I was learning new skills and adapting to my "new normal" after the transplant. I tolerated and managed my questionable stamina and fatigue, trusting it would eventually pass. I enjoyed my students and loved being able to teach again, relishing every moment I was in the classroom or engaged with students. I didn't miss a day those first eight weeks, and I only left work early a few times. Working inside my current abilities was still a challenge, largely because I'd never experienced serious limitations before the transplant. But I started realizing my deficiencies were survivable.

Learning who I was now and what I could and couldn't do was immensely helpful in accepting my change in health status and impending retirement. My return to Oakton allowed me to end my career on my own terms and in a positive way. I wouldn't have missed finishing my teaching career in this way for anything in the world (except perhaps perfect original kidneys). I had such appreciation and gratitude for being at Oakton. What a wonderful place to work.

Early in March, during Oakton's spring break, Audrey and I went to Tucson, Arizona, to visit our dear friends, Alan and Patty Rubin, who spent winters there. We were joined by our other wonderful friends Smokey and Elaine Daniels. We relaxed and enjoyed the incomparable company and the gorgeous spring desert. It was a welcome respite from the world of work and routine. We laughed, ate wonderful meals, and absorbed the warm Arizona sun. It couldn't have been better. I even played golf twice and hiked in the desert. Mostly we relaxed. Once again, the support, kindness, and generosity of friends enhanced my life and filled my heart with joy and goodness.

We returned to an unseasonably warm Chicago and the homestretch of my career. The gravity of retiring was sinking in: I felt simultaneously happy and sad. I was certain that retiring, especially in light of my physical condition, was the right thing to do, but I also felt the heaviness of ending a career I dearly loved. Every day became a gift to relish and appreciate. I had a strange convergence of experiences. Three dynamics were operating simultaneously: acute mindfulness of my energy and stamina; grief over the loss of a career I loved; and the thrill of spending time with my students and colleagues for the last time.

One afternoon in mid-March, toward the end of my "last" spring break, I walked downstairs to my office and started typing the beginnings of this book. Although those earliest efforts were ramblings that chronicled what had happened (which would be revised and edited countless times), capturing ideas on the page after having talked about it for months created a bit of momentum. Reflecting on the act of starting to write, something I had thought about often, illuminated the connection between talking about a goal or desire and making it "real" and tangible. The more I talked about writing a book, the more I felt obligated to do so. In fact, the writing had actually commenced in my head during our journey to Tucson.

On the plane to Arizona I had a reality check about my level of emotional healing while attempting to read a book. Emily had met Suzanne F. Ruff, author of *The Reluctant Donor*, while attending fundraiser training at the PKD Foundation. Emily described my plans to write a book, and Suzanne graciously sent me a copy of her book about donating a kidney to her sister. Audrey read *The Reluctant Donor* first and raved about it, passing it on to my sister Roseann, who also enjoyed it. To my knowledge, *The Reluctant Donor* is the only book published about being a donor for a PKD patient and the effects of this disease on a family. When I started to read it on the flight to Tucson, I burst into tears before finishing the first page. I was shocked by my response. Apparently, I had some more healing to do before I was emotionally ready to delve into a kidney-transplant story five months after my own transplant. As I recovered from my mini catharsis, I concluded it was better to wait until I wrote my own story before I read someone else's. Write first, read later.

Physical health returned far in advance of my emotional, psychological, and spiritual healing. I was back at work. And, yes, my doctors were pleased with my progress, particularly, my labs. But I still had some inner work to do to recover from the trauma of my experience. In order to make peace with my loss of health and new condition, I had to grieve. One of the key aspects of grieving is a realistic assessment of what was lost, meaning not demonizing or idealizing, but rather seeing the reality of the situation. My understanding of this aspect of grieving comes from Harvard psychologist Samuel Osherson's book, *Finding Our Fathers*. (I used this book in my men's psychology class to explore the healing of men's father wounds. Osherson also spoke at our Men's Day at Oakton in the 1980s.) Grieving was the path to healing, to wholeness. Processing all that had taken place would simply take time. Searching for truth requires time and patience. There are no shortcuts. The adage "Time heals," was certainly true for me.

After the Arizona trip, I stayed with my work-then-rest pattern. The rule of doing one thing a day held true. My lack of stamina was my primary concern. In this new normal I could work, go to the gym, socialize, or even play golf. But now "normal" was limited. This adjustment bothered me; it was a loss. I hoped I would eventually reset to my previous level of energy and stamina. I never really did.

Come late March and April, while I wrestled with the issues of stamina and grieving, Audrey bottomed out. She got very sick and was forced to take a week off from work, which was frowned upon at her job and added to her stress. At first we thought it was the flu or an infection of some sort. When her health didn't improve, she finally went to the doctor. Audrey had infectious colitis, a stress-related illness. She was very ill and immobilized. It had likely been in her system for months. Finally, with a vengeance, it emerged and overtook her. Although she was a warrior, she succumbed to the strain of everything she'd been through—physically and emotionally—for the past sixteen months. She was lucky it wasn't more serious. It forced her to slow down and press the reset button. Relief was in sight though—we were returning to Florida in about four weeks.

Audrey recovered slowly. What she needed most was rest and a release from the responsibility of caring for another person 24/7. She needed to be taken care of. She accomplished the first two by lying on the couch. Happily, by this point, I was able to step up and be a caretaker, at least in a limited way. My "can do" list was growing. I went grocery shopping, prepared simple meals, and got her the things she needed while she recuperated. I enjoyed being a giver and not a taker. It felt like a small repayment for all she'd done and been through for the past year and a half. I teased her that because I'd taken care of her for about a week, we were "even." Occasionally she smiled at the silliness of my comment; other times, she looked at me confused— like I had two heads or a "case of the stupids."

Even though my daily activities were managed, I was mentally weary. Like a battery losing its juice, I eventually lost my giddyup. Perhaps it was the cumulative fatigue or the emotional intensity of ending my recovery as my career came to a close. Who knew saying good-bye was so exhausting? The strain hit me as April ended. Even though I persevered, I was forced to take a couple of days off. I think I had the flu and a cold. Whatever it was, I could barely get off the couch. My perfect attendance record was ruined. Alas.

Curiously, all this was happening around the six-month mark of the transplant. The Transplant Clinic staff had told me how good I was going to feel at six months. With expectations high, I couldn't wait to reach the magic number. I thought my recovery would be complete. My improvement was obvious physically in terms of energy and strength. Working was proof of that, right? But I didn't feel "great." Stamina was missing. Not wanting to complain, I trudged on. My disappointment made me feel guilty. For the first time, I thought maybe I was doing too much. Perhaps going back to work wasn't so smart. The hidden cost of redirecting my energy from recovering to work came due, and I needed to readjust and find a new balance.

I limped through the last weeks, doing too much after coming back too soon. Determination and grit got me through it, but I struggled mightily. I put one foot in front of the other, a familiar routine. In addition to teaching my classes and dealing with student issues, I was cleaning out my office, discarding thirty-one years of accumulated stuff. I threw away an endless number of folders and packed dozens of boxes. In retrospect, throwing away all that stuff was symbolic of my forthcoming life change—get ready for the new by discarding the old. The packing didn't end until the final minutes of my last day on campus. Surely, in part, it was an unconscious resistance to retiring. I gave away most of the boxes, but I took a few home. They remained in my basement untouched for fifteen months.

I graded papers and posted grades for the last time. I had made it to the finish line. The semester culminated in the final commencement I'd attend at Oakton, the final installment in a series of "last times" that had been going on for a year. I was a reluctant attendee until I saw one of my former students cross the stage. My ambivalent attitude adjusted as tears filled my eyes. I realized I was graduating too.

Our plan was to leave the day after graduation for Florida. And somehow we managed it. As it had in January, Florida worked its magic. Energy returned. Not the limited energy of winter and spring, but the energy I'd known before I went into renal failure. Resting, relaxing, and having fun for ten days in Florida was recuperative. The first thing I noticed was that I slept better and longer. Mindful of our activities and pace, we slowed way down. It worked for the both of us.

It took eight months, not six, before I turned the corner. Consistently I felt like my old self again. I had energy and sufficient stamina. As each day brought me nearer to how I remembered feeling, I wondered if there were a chance I'd regain my full health. I learned the body works in its own way and at its own pace. It's impossible to predict how an individual will respond to a disease and its treatment. I reflected on just how human we all are—patients and caretakers.

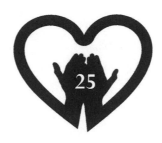

ENDINGS AND BEGINNINGS

You say good-bye and I say hello. Hello. Hello.

—THE BEATLES

Commencement at Oakton and our Florida trip that spring signaled the end of my career was extremely close at hand. Work as I knew it was all but over, and retirement was about to commence. Six days at Oakton, spread over the next three weeks, was all that remained. Fortunately, those final days were "call" days, which for counselors means being available for any emergency or student crisis that might occur. I intended to spend my free time packing and saying farewell.

Completing a thirty-four-year career was difficult emotionally. It created a multitude of strange feelings: confusion, loss, detachment, and sense of being carefree. On those final days, I would arrive at my office, do a little paperwork, work on emptying out my files, and pack whatever didn't get tossed into the recycling bin or the garbage can. The monotony was wearing. The only interruptions were when a colleague or student stopped by to chat or say good-bye. I strategically planned several lunches with close friends to ensure closure and fight the boredom.

My last two days were unexpectedly interrupted by a handful of student "crises." I capped off my career doing what I was there in the first place to do—counseling. Although it made the time for packing tighter, I was pleased I had these last few student contacts. It was grounding. But these interventions did create the one thing I hated most about being on call—paperwork. Forms had to be filled out and referrals made. All in a day's work, I figured . . . and all for the last time.

My last day was strange, comical, and, oddly, an appropriate ending to my career. With packing still to do, the situation almost got out of control. A last-minute lunch was interrupted by a call from the secretary. My services were required—a student needed help. Off I went. Ironically, it was one of the few times I'd ever been called in for a student emergency when off campus in my thirty-one years at Oakton. Although it was a minor problem, it took a few hours to resolve. I felt the clock ticking.

I wanted to say farewell to Joi Smith, the vice president of student affairs, and Peg Lee, the president of the college. Scurrying about, I completed those final good-byes. After that somewhat frantic rushing around, I got back to my office to find my buddies Cary and Paul waiting. The plan was to meet half a dozen friends for a drink. When asked months earlier how I wanted things to go, I said I didn't want to leave on my last day alone and in total anonymity, walking out the door with a box in my hands. To prevent this dismal end, they walked me out the door. Carrying my personal items and pulling a cart with boxes, my "last walk," felt discombobulating.

I went to get my car. I couldn't find it. There I was, in my last moments at the college, roaming around the faculty parking lot—bewildered, frustrated, and amused. After nearly ten minutes, I remembered I'd parked in the guest lot because of the student emergency. Initially embarrassed at my forgetfulness, I later recognized my experience was based on what Laurence Gonzales—in his book *Deep Survival*—calls "emotional memory," relying on the emotions of a previous experience to direct your behavior. I'd parked in the faculty lot for thirty-plus years. Why wouldn't I expect to find my car there on my last day?

Cary, Paul, and I laughed. They had some great new teasing material to deploy in the days, weeks, and even months to come. We finally made it to the bar where more friends were waiting. What a terrific punctuation mark on my career. I felt satisfied.

Unofficially, my retirement started on June 13, 2012; the official date was July 1, 2012. I was ready. Perhaps if the last year and a half had been different, I might've had second thoughts. But in my heart, I knew this part of my life was over. Moving forward, I was feeling healthy and complete in my career. I did worry about what would become of me post-transplant. Life would never be the same. All remnants of the invulnerability that comes with *not* having serious health problems were gone. Aging wouldn't be done in the usual fashion. For example, my risk of skin cancer is now sixty-five times greater than the average person. Dr. Becker had clearly indicated that it wasn't *if* I'd get skin cancer, but *when*. Her prediction was daunting. This increased risk exemplifies the transformation that took place in my life and how the future would be influenced by it. The task was to live as normal a life as possible, regardless of the inevitable changes. At this point in my recovery—eight months—I saw my circumstance as a challenge rather than a problem. Other than a larger waist and a bulge on the right side of my abdomen, there were no telltale signs of what I'd experienced. Unless I told someone I'd had a kidney transplant, they were unlikely to suspect that was the case.

As my physical capacities increased, I grew more confident that not only was I going to survive, but I was going to live an essentially normal life (with some exceptions). Acutely conscious of how my current life was a gift, my prevailing attitude was fueled by gratitude for the good fortune of my recovery thus far. Rather than speculating about why I was the recipient of the series of miracles that had brought me to this point (although this never entirely subsides), I focused on what I might do as a result of such good fortune. *Given a second chance at living, what can I accomplish? How can I pay it forward so another person might benefit from my experience?* My first answer was writing this book. Maybe other PKD patients needing a transplant and their families might learn from my experience.

On my first unofficial day of retirement, I knew the decision to retire was the right one. I planned to move forward with my life in earnest, with no second thoughts. I was as ready as I could be. But my lofty thoughts were tempered by the practicalities of household responsibilities and other obligations. I was going to have to integrate it all into a functional whole. At the top of my priorities was trying to make Audrey's life a little easier, finding ways to pay back some of what she'd done. I knew realistically that recompense was never totally possible, but perhaps my efforts would be appreciated and her load lightened. Audrey was in no way resentful of my retirement; she was committed to her job for another year and a half. I affectionately teased her that going to the grocery store and cooking a few dinners actually put her back in the red and she owed me again. She only chuckled a bit.

Bret came to town at the end of June to have his six-month postoperative checkup—in his case, it was accomplished a little late at eight months. We knew through our conversations with Emily that he'd complained earlier about some abdominal pain. Consequently, Audrey and I were extremely relieved he was finally getting checked out. His ten-month-old baby daughter, Hadley, and his girlfriend, Melissa Fergeson, came with him. We looked forward to showing them Chicago and playing with Hadley. Bret's follow-up exam went well. The pain in his abdomen, which we thought might be a surgical hernia, turned out to be the muscle over a stitch that hadn't fully healed. All he had to do was exercise to strengthen the area. Good news.

Audrey threw me a surprise retirement party during Bret's visit. It was also an opportunity for my friends, who had loved and admired him from afar, to meet and thank him. He was graciously welcomed and treated like the hero he was. This surprise event punctuated my retirement saga and signaled the start of my new life.

Summer, with its joys and splendors, took over the next two months. But my regular clinic visits remained. With my labs coming in as "perfect," I was able to be very active and enjoy my return to health. "Perfect" was the superlative the UChicago Transplant Clinic nurses (Jo, Mary Beth, and Roseann) used when they called me with my lab results. How joyful it was to hear that word regarding my kidney function. I often got a little teary-eyed as the sound of it resonated through me. Thankfully, my clinic visits grew shorter, with more time in between. They largely consisted of getting lab work done and the staff asking how I was and if I had any questions. After a few minutes, the appointment ended. I started seriously considering that my appointment on September 12, the eleven-month anniversary, would be my last follow-up at the clinic.

Mulling over this possibility, I realized my journey was concluding. My twenty-two-month odyssey was in its final weeks. My musings were often followed by uncertainty. Questions flew around in my head: *Am I ready? Am I healthy?* I wanted to move on and be done with this part of my life, but at the same time my connection with the Transplant Clinic—the nurses and doctors—was an anchor that provided comfort and safety. But one fact was clear: my association with the clinic was going to end at the twelve-month anniversary because of the insurance coverage. I needed to prepare myself for that part of the journey to end.

Finishing at the clinic would be a graduation, a commencement. With their blessing bestowed, I could move on to my independence. With my new kidney firmly attached and functioning perfectly, I was free to live my life however I chose. Amazing! How often does this type of situation occur in an adult life? Rarely. Instead of concentrating on recovering, I shifted my focus to living—in all its scary, daunting, and wildly exciting facets—with the gift I'd been given.

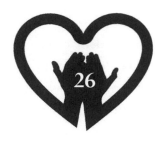

RETURNING TO WELLNESS

Life is a series of collisions with the future; it is not the sum of
what we have been, but what we yearn to be.

—José Ortega y Gasset

As my recovery progressed and I got stronger, I mentally committed to living my life as if I'd never had a kidney transplant. To my way of thinking, that meant attempting to do everything I'd done previously. My only limits were fatigue and physical shortcomings. I tested my progress against my "normal" of years past. I earnestly sought to identify my strengths or deficits in terms of my overall recovery.

Armed with this mind-set, I committed to a physical routine and a healthy lifestyle. I went to the gym at least three times per week, attempting to increase my endurance, strength, and flexibility. My initial exercise routine included thirty-three minutes on the elliptical, walking to cool down, hitting the Nautilus machines to build back muscle mass lost during my recuperation, and then stretching for ten to fifteen minutes. All told, it took an hour and fifteen minutes, a challenging commitment. Even though my endurance increased, I couldn't maintain this degree of effort. It was too exhausting. So I adapted and let how I felt determine which exercises I did and for how long.

In addition to regular trips to the gym, I walked with Audrey and played golf, alternating walking or taking a cart. I wanted to be physically active six days a week. Fatigue forced me to cut back to five days. My body simply tired out and my muscles ached. Playing golf in the oppressive heat depleted my energy and stamina. Because I so much wanted to be the Greg I used to be, these setbacks frustrated and discouraged me.

I operated at about an 8 to 10 percent deficit from where I'd been prior to renal failure. My stamina improved, but my pace didn't. As I approached the one-year anniversary, I was still establishing my new normal physically. I harbored the belief that I could return to and maybe even surpass my previous physical capacity, even though I was almost two years older and about to turn sixty-one. Now I realize this was foolhardy and unnecessary.

During the summer I relearned that recovery wasn't only about the physical, even as I focused on that side because it was tangible and measurable. As I was zealously working to gain endurance, I was struggling cognitively. The recognizable loss of some mental acuity was disturbing, and it threatened to be the most severe limitation I'd faced. I discovered that while playing golf, my ability to concentrate would sometimes fail me. The best example of my condition was that midway through a round of golf, I would "space out" and lose my ability to focus on the activity at hand. My mind and body weren't connected. This loss of focus was distressing. I was unable to quickly reset; it could last thirty or even sixty minutes. The gaps persisted despite my efforts to counteract them.

I hadn't experienced similar lapses during other activities. I wrote for hours at a time without experiencing a mental letdown. Only when my actions required both mental concentration and physical effort did these cognitive lapses occur. My loss of mental acuity was the most troubling of any of the challenges I'd encountered thus far.

Earlier in my recovery I worked through memory gaps and forgetfulness—usually while I was teaching or driving. What alarmed me the most now was that my deficits persisted despite my efforts to repel them. I felt worried by this ongoing situation that threatened to impact essential areas of my life. When I shared my dilemma with friends, most of them laughed and said, "Welcome to your sixties." I was reluctant to believe it was solely about my age. I maintained it was a postsurgical issue. Feelings of vulnerability were often present and occasionally overwhelmed me. I was scared.

The gaps in concentration continued all summer and into the fall. I eventually learned that these episodes correlated with my fatigue level. The quicker I tired, the more likely I was to have a lapse. I was unable to completely avoid or offset the dips in energy that led to my spacing out, but it did improve when I cut back the frequency and intensity of activities. Less was, in fact, more. I continued to lag behind where I was two years earlier. Deficits in my levels of stamina and energy persisted. I did, however, learn over time to accept the current reality and modify my expectations.

Despite continuing to "normalize" my life, bouts of vulnerability and anxiety persisted. It was particularly present when I drove. I nervously braked whenever a car came to an intersection, scaring whoever was with me. This struggle decreased over time, but it didn't extinguish completely for a long time. Socially, I resisted being around crowds of people, in which I could feel constricted or claustrophobic. My conflict was best illustrated by a tiff Audrey and I had over attending a Bruce Springsteen concert at Wrigley Field in early September 2012. Audrey wanted to attend; I balked at the suggestion. I wasn't ready for a rock concert where the alcohol-infused intensity of fans and the mind-numbing, incredibly loud music seemed threatening. My fear was a carry-over of the postsurgery vulnerability I experienced after the transplant. Feeling guilty about what a devoted caretaker she'd been, I unfortunately left the door open to going. The conflict reemerged right before the concert. We had a horrible argument, something we rarely did. But considering what we went through for twenty months, perhaps we needed an excuse to release some pent-up emotion and frustration. We had a Vesuvius moment. The discharge of tension, albeit necessary, was disturbing.

Our heated debate got me wondering about the role of vulnerability in my life and how ever-present and prominent it was, whether it was conscious or unconscious. Getting older increased my sense of helplessness and fear. As my physical strength and capacities decreased and my mental abilities skipped a beat, my confidence waned. I doubted my readiness to escape from a threatening situation. I felt overwhelmed much more quickly. End-stage renal disease followed by a serious surgery and long-term recovery combined to fuel my lack of confidence and exacerbate my fear and sense of helplessness. I was more hesitant and cautious. Although improving, I worried about my life becoming more restricted. These were definitely new, post-transplant issues for me. But one thing, one attitude, was clear in the face of feeling vulnerable: persist, struggle, and try to be brave.

I thought of myself as a risk taker who was willing to take reasonable chances. Previously I saw myself as mentally sharp and physically strong enough to overcome the challenges life presented. But the world I was currently living felt like it was closing in, becoming more imposing and consequently more intimidating. I no longer trusted that my physical strength or mental capacity allowed me to respond to a threat, real or perceived, in a fashion that could get me out of harm's way. The reality of aging and recuperating from surgery resulted in my acting more cautious than ever before. Consequently, going to a rock concert wasn't on my playlist—even if it meant disappointing Audrey.

In my current state of mind, I felt diminished as a person, and my fear and vulnerability were exposed. Awareness of what I was going through emotionally was helpful. Owning how I was feeling was liberating. I learned to recognize what I'm experiencing in real time—and naming what's making me feel vulnerable helps decrease its intensity and duration. This path of acknowledgment led to quicker resolution and, most importantly, to acceptance—both of my mental state and how I was aging. I staunchly believe accepting one's limitations while persisting and carrying on is emancipating. Not judging myself by unreasonable standards paved the way to patience, acceptance, and improvement—my fears and sense of vulnerability decreased.

Despite my other struggles, my labs remained consistently excellent. My one-year transplant anniversary loomed large on the horizon. It was difficult to comprehend that I had come so far. Time, paradoxically, had passed quickly and slowly. Evidently, I successfully navigated the most treacherous period—when I was at the greatest risk of rejection. Thinking about my impending transition away from being a patient at the Transplant Clinic was simultaneously exhilarating and intimidating. I started viewing all that had happened to me in the rearview mirror. Because I felt safe under the watchful eyes of the clinic staff, separating from them was a bit intimidating. I was leaving the nest.

Life was charging forward, more so than ever before. The recovery phase had moved to its natural conclusion, and I was enthusiastic about the future. But I was left with a head-spinning question. *Who is Greg with a new kidney anyway?* Although I would always be a kidney-transplant patient, it wasn't useful to only self-identify that way. This adjustment coincided with my new life in retirement, a transition that calls for a redefinition of one's self and life. My anxiety slowly subsided and was replaced by gratitude for surviving my health crisis.

My grateful meter reached new heights on August 18, 2012. Sarah had a baby, Cybele Beatrix. We became grandparents. It felt significant that Cybele's arrival coincided with the conclusion of my yearlong recovery. New life begets new life and cultivates it. Words can't describe the joy and elation Audrey and I felt. Cybele's arrival highlighted the circle-of-life saga my family and I were participating in.

Gratitude. My life was literally overflowing with it. Beginning with my sister and cousins and friends offering to donate a kidney, continuing with Bret's life-giving gift, and now culminating in the birth of a new generation. Babies are intrinsically life-affirming. A baby's presence fills everyone with hope and optimism. The ecstasy we felt stamped out any lingering hurt, pessimism, despair, anxiety, or worry. Joy shined so brightly around Cybele; she bathed us all in a sense of wholeness and worth. And she was perfectly healthy, the antithesis of me. From the first few hours through the following days, weeks, and months, I felt restored.

Cybele's birth, my return to good health, and the one-year anniversary of my transplant surgery coalesced to fill me with wonder. My story had come full circle. My small saga was dwarfed by the bigger story of new life.

Visiting Cybele and her parents in DC illuminated the past twenty months in new ways. Being in her presence was amazing. As babies tend to do, Cybele became the center of attention. As the days passed, we sat and looked at her and smiled. Sarah is a wonderful mother. Seeing our daughter with her new child and how she looked at Cybele was an unexpected pleasure. We couldn't help but remember how thirty-six years ago we'd looked at her in the same way. Humans are engrossed by their children. The way a parent looks at a new child is a unique and life-giving gaze. It communicates love, affirmation, care, commitment, strength, and joy all at once.

Sarah becoming a mom and assuming the role so effortlessly affirmed how we felt about her as our daughter. We'd come full circle with our firstborn grandchild. It confirmed our role as parents and added a new one—grandparents. Grammy and Grampy. Sarah was moving on to bigger and better things, and so were we.

We left DC full. Our lives were richer now than they had ever been. Cybele's fresh, new life and my figurative new life made the future bright—and filled it with optimism and opportunity. A future so rich with possibility was a stark contrast to twenty months earlier when I was filled with loss and fear. Then I had to constrict and close down to protect myself, and now I was choosing to open up to possibility and growth. How my life evolved in such a way was unclear. Pain, fear, and loss were replaced by love, light, and life. Although understanding the reasons was elusive, acceptance was not. I chose simply to relish what I'd learned along the way.

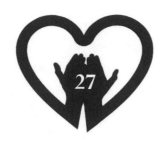

WINDING DOWN, WRAPPING UP, MOVING ON

*All the art of living lies in a fine mingling of letting go
and holding on.*

—HAVELOCK ELLIS

On September 12, 2012, I went to what turned out to be my last visit at the Transplant Clinic. It started as an ordinary visit, something I'd done a dozen times before. The alarm sounded at 5:50 a.m. I arose sleepily and stumbled into the bathroom for a shower, the start of my morning routine. Then it was down to the kitchen for a snack of toast with a little turkey for protein and some black coffee. I sat and stared at the TV for a half hour before I started my drive.

I saw an awe-inspiring sunrise over Lake Michigan, echoing the one we'd seen on the way to my first post-transplant visit. *How stunning,* I thought, *the sunrise never fails to impress. No wonder it's a universal symbol for optimism.* No matter how good I felt, I always wondered on the way to my clinic visits what would be in store for me today. Would it be thumbs up or down? Good news or bad? More tests or not?

Atypically the traffic was light, and I made it in record time—forty-four minutes, a personal best. I was so early that I was first in line for the hospital's valet parkers. That had never happened before. I was also the first patient of the day. Off I went to have my kidney-function labs done and then back to the clinic waiting area to be seen by the nurses and doctor. The typical wait, which could push two hours, was only five minutes. I was weighed and my blood pressure was taken. Nothing was out of the ordinary. After being escorted to the exam room, I settled in for the medical staff to arrive. Instead of the normal thirty minutes of alone time, Jo, the nurse, arrived in ten. Was this unusual series of fortuitous events this day merely random occurrences or noteworthy of something else? While reviewing the lab results, she commented that I was eleven months from surgery. The conversation turned from my results to a discussion about starting to see my regular primary care physician and nephrologist. Curiously, I'd received a call just the day before from the hospital's insurance department informing me that the referral from my doctor had expired in August. My day and clinic visit were now clearly out of the ordinary. Change was afoot.

With sterling lab numbers again and no cause of concern moving forward, Jo and I concluded that my present relationship with the Transplant Clinic could end. We would part ways for now, and my treatment would shift to my regular doctors. *Hallelujah!* The department fellow agreed and the staff nephrologist, Dr. Cunningham, concurred. I was done. I had anticipated my time at the clinic ending, but the realization that the clinic part of my saga was complete finally registered in my brain when Cunningham (the opinion that really mattered) repeated the same message for the third time.

My finale at the clinic was unceremonious—even blasé. No fanfare, no music, and no prize. None were necessary. My health and a beautifully functioning kidney were reward enough. I left in excellent condition and feeling great. The medical staff had been brilliant. Even to the last moment, they were happy for me, supportive and encouraging as I walked out the door. My last visit was over by nine o'clock, another record. I wouldn't return for a follow-up visit, barring an emergency, for a full year.

The magnitude of what just transpired didn't hit me until I was in the lobby waiting for my car. Looking around the waiting area and watching the patients and medical personnel scurry about, I was struck by how incredibly busy this place was—the exact same thought I'd had in February 2011 when I attended the orientation session. I was filled with reverence back then and still felt amazed as my adventure culminated now. *How impressive,* I reflected as I stood there trembling, *this place and the people here saved my life. Incredible.* I was having a moment.

As I drove away from the hospital for the last time, I called Audrey, but we talked only briefly. It was good to hear her voice. I was in urgent need of a reality check. We chatted for few moments, maybe sixty seconds. The demands of her job wouldn't be denied. I hoped her voice would anchor me so I could drive home. It didn't work.

A few miles from the hospital, the sheer emotion of my separation and closure from the clinic overcame me. I felt overwhelmed, and then . . . *wham!* I started sobbing. I pulled the car over to prevent an accident. I was astonished by what had transpired in the past twenty-two months. I was on the other side of a miracle. I was given a new life by the generosity of a stranger. I emerged, intact, from an ordeal that changed not just my daily circumstances, but my life in a holistic sense. All of these thoughts and feelings exploded simultaneously.

I hadn't anticipated such a profound, emotion-filled reaction. I expected to be happy and relieved about being released from the clinic, but not at this intensity. But we don't get forewarned, do we? No email or telephone call alerts us of impending emotional overload. As my tears slowed and an evenness of breathing returned, my head cleared. It was time to finish the drive home. In the ever-present traffic on Lake Shore Drive, I struggled to stay in the moment. This experience was an epiphany for me. Being behind the wheel was the only thing keeping me tethered to reality. I only slipped into the space between worlds for milliseconds at a time.

After getting a snack and a grande latte at Starbucks, hoping it would ground me, I went home and settled in to text my family and Bret: "Family, Had last clinic visit this morning at UChicago—all is good. What an amazing year it's been. Who knew I'd be at this point feeling so good and being so healthy. Very emotional. Cried on the drive home. Thank you, Bret, for your big heart and precious kidney. Thank you, family, for all you did and continue to do. Love you all, G."

The tears flowed all the while I pecked on those little phone keys. Those intense and raw moments validate our humanity—and, wow, was I feeling mine. *Another blessing, another gift out of nowhere. Well, actually, out of someone.* My astounding odyssey had reached its natural conclusion, but my saga continued.

Completing my work at the clinic signaled the end of my recovery reality. I reached a threshold of sorts. I would no longer be defined as a recovering kidney-transplant patient. A new identity was in order as I approached the one-year anniversary date: October 12, 2012, one month away. I was a kidney transplant patient, but my recovery was now complete.

September marched ahead alongside my new awareness that life was resetting. New coordinates for where I would go from here needed to be set. The rhythms of things were shifting—some remained familiar, others felt vastly different. I contacted my regular doctors and scheduled appointments. As good as the medical staff was at the Transplant Clinic, returning to the doctors who had kept me healthy for years delighted me. There was comfort and satisfaction in seeing them again. I was done with the long drive to Hyde Park for checkups. *Yes!* Most importantly, returning to the familiar meant that I was healthy—no lingering severe or threatening problems from the transplant surgery. And it was exhilarating. I crossed the threshold of survival and was secure—at least for the foreseeable future. Life and I were moving on.

Next up was our trip to Cleveland for a PKD walk and fundraiser Emily had planned. Drawing on her remarkable organizational skills, she'd become a fundraiser for the Northeast Ohio PKD Foundation chapter. When she expressed an interest in participating, she was asked to take charge of the annual fundraising walk. With a natural passion and personal interest, she committed her time and skills to raising money for PKD research. Faithfully, throughout the winter she drove to various meeting places in northeast Ohio to garner support for the big event. She met tirelessly with local hospitals, including the Cleveland Clinic and the University Hospitals at Case Medical Complex (affiliated with Case Western Reserve University). She even visited local dialysis centers to get donations and solicit support.

Emily's actions, passion, and commitment inspired me, both as a parent and recent transplant patient. I was proud of how she took action. As parents, we always *love* our children. It's the natural and right thing to do. But also as parents, we don't always *like* our children, especially when they're surly, foolish, or belligerent. These observations translated into my belief that a true test of parenting is if you not only *love* your children when they're grown up, but also *like* the person they've become. If they're good human beings who participate in their own lives and make a contribution to the greater good, I concluded, Audrey and I must have done something well as parents. Emily supported that theory, and I *loved* and *liked* her as I observed the person she was.

The PKD walk was immensely successful. Emily doubled the funds raised the previous year and surpassed her goal by five thousand dollars. The total amount collected to help find a cure for polycystic kidney disease was more than thirty thousand dollars. Amazing. Close to two hundred people walked to support the PKD Foundation, including Bret and his family members, other friends of Emily and Terry, and their family members as well. After the walk, Emily and Terry hosted a backyard barbecue to celebrate the event's success. The gathering also served as a housewarming for their new home. Sarah and Chris came all the way from DC and our new granddaughter, Cybele, was the guest of honor.

One downside of all the festivities—hundreds of pictures were taken. I looked unmistakably like a kidney transplant patient. In my eyes, I looked huge. Although I hadn't gained weight, largely due to exercise and diet, the additional bulk of my old, enlarged kidneys was obvious. Steroids added a puffy, buttery roll around my abdomen. PKD-afflicted kidneys can weigh up to twenty pounds, but worse than the added weight, they push everything forward. My sudden self-consciousness was a shock. Even though I'd never considered myself vain, that day I reacted like someone obsessed by vanity. People surrounded me, most of them young and attractive. I wanted to hide. I wanted to leave. Later when I saw myself in the photos, I felt terrible, deformed even.

Self-pity was a dilemma. I knew self-acceptance was essential. There was little I could do to fix the problem of my physical appearance. The doctors wouldn't remove the old kidneys unless there was a significant medical reason to do so. Vanity wasn't a sufficient reason. And, realistically, I didn't want the risk and pain of yet another abdominal procedure that would render me incapacitated for months.

I often thought about the hump on my right lower abdomen, largely in the context of my pants size increasing by four inches. I discarded almost every pair of pants I'd owned prior to the transplant surgery and slowly replaced them. I avoided looking at myself in the mirror. I participated in my own fantasy of being thinner, feeling far skinnier on the inside. This experience revealed my beliefs about being overweight and body image.

My struggle was only fueled by shame and embarrassment about worrying about such trivial things. I had survived a harrowing experience. I was healthy. Harsh self-judgment about my weight and how I looked seemed shallow. It seemed petty. I felt bad, and then felt bad about feeling bad. I was out of sorts and out of whack. I was oh so human. A perfect kidney didn't make me a perfect person.

Fortunately, when we left Cleveland, my self-pitying abated. I started rethinking my shame and started to accept myself. How I felt about how I thought I looked began to lose its power. My overactive, self-critical mind was resetting to a saner and more normal place. I realized I could live with how I looked and accept the death of my vanity. After all the gifts I'd been given, not looking slim, trim, and beautiful was a small price to pay. The alternatives—being sick, disabled, limited, or even dead—were far worse. Still, it was painful to examine a part of me I didn't like or accept. I'd touched a vulnerable and tender place in my psyche, and another of my human weaknesses was revealed to me. My wish was to have it all: to be healthy and unscathed by the illness, transplant, and recovery. That was an impossible fantasy. Couple this awareness with getting older and the normal loss and decline of one's physical appearance and abilities, and you get a strong dose of reality smacking you in the face.

Though I came around to a more positive outlook, my ugly feelings revisited me from time to time. Emancipation from my irrational thinking was a process of ups and downs, peaks and valleys. I couldn't escape my human flaws, but I was confident that as time passed I'd accept myself for who I was now. My gratitude helped me do that.

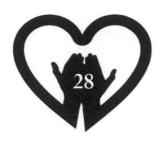

HAPPY ANNIVERSARY, HAPPY ANNIVERSARY, HAAAAAPPY ANNIVERSARY!

A life spent making mistakes is not only more honorable, but more useful than a life spent doing nothing.

—George Bernard Shaw

My focus turned to my rapidly approaching anniversary date: October 12. I savored the importance of the one-year mark. I envisioned this benchmark as a time of triumph and celebration. It seemed strange to think a whole year had passed since that auspicious day. So much had happened. Getting a kidney transplant was something I'd consciously and unconsciously dreaded—even agonized about— since early adolescence. Now, at the one-year point, I could look back and understand that I'd survived this dreaded and perilous journey virtually unscathed.

I had a powerful sense of satisfaction. Being forced to confront my worst fears, surviving the threat, and coming out the other side humbled me and enhanced my sense of who I'd become. Acknowledging the fine line between survival and accomplishment, I felt I'd not only endured, but also flourished. I'd earned new insights, a broader perspective of life and living. The volume had been turned up on life. With the distance of time, I could see my transplant journey as a gift that truly enriched my life.

It was an unexpected discovery. I never thought a terrible disease, major surgery, and months of recovery would result in such a positive attitude. I wanted to yell "Thank you!" to the heavens. How amazing that my body essentially failed me, but the result was an opening of new spiritual and emotional aspects of my life. Life was simply not the same anymore. My new consciousness offered a newfound freedom that allowed me to transcend some of the limitations of my body. I wanted to cultivate my new perspective. The human body inevitably falters and eventually fails, but contained in that physical failure is an opportunity to see life differently. Rather than being dominated by measuring physical prowess and its limits, I could choose to examine other aspects of my life. Unexpectedly, transplant surgery ignited a process of addition rather than subtraction in my life.

Although the ability to see life from a different perspective (i.e., to *reframe* one's experience) empowers and liberates, I didn't want to wax philosophical all the time. I decided that living in a physical world is essential, and it requires keeping both feet on the ground. I needed to be realistic about my health. My body and its condition anchor me to the physical world. I'm still at risk. Numerous things could go wrong, and other medical issues could develop. The risk of diabetes and skin cancer are among the top concerns. As I age, the long-term effects of taking immunosuppressant medications will have a negative impact. Taking a different perspective helps, but the physical reality is inescapably present. Still, I find it fun and enjoyable to *play* with these ideas in my head and heart. The Andean shamans call this *sacred play*, meaning to engage life with a beginner's mind and curiosity that allows an openness to what can be discovered through engagement rather than the inertia of old patterns.

With my transplant anniversary imminent, I felt resolute and strong, even triumphant. There was much to be thankful for and to celebrate. For the moment, victory was mine. I survived the most threatening ordeal of my life and was still standing. I wanted to mark this milestone. I wanted to use the power of the moment to propel me forward and strengthen my resolve to a more expansive approach to living. I wanted to harness the strength I garnered from meeting the kidney crisis to face the challenges that certainly awaited me in the future. I wanted to be available to the present. And the current moment was truly a present, a gift—glorious, beautiful, and gratifying.

Gratitude for my journey is always heightened by seeing Bret. Being around him and enjoying him interacting with his daughter, Hadley, only deepens what I thought was an already bottomless well of appreciation for his gift. Even years later, I feel deeply humble in his presence. Oddly, I still find it difficult to talk to him, as if the right words are unavailable. I don't know what to say other than to continually thank him. Audrey connects easily with Bret and has often acted as a conduit between the two of us. Bret is more comfortable with her, I think, because he also feels the ever-present intensity between us. Audrey bridges that space and makes our encounters easier. Bret is the epicenter of my transplant experience; it all comes back to his generosity. His humility deepens the meaning of my experience and illustrates how quiet, unassuming people have powerful and profound effects on others.

To celebrate the actual anniversary, Audrey and I traveled to Bar Harbor, Maine, and then to Washington, DC, to visit Sarah, Chris, and Cybele again. Going to the East Coast for the autumn colors was a lifelong wish that my teaching schedule had precluded. We couldn't have picked two better destinations. Acadia National Park in Maine is stunning, and our new granddaughter was in DC. Maine's beautiful coast reminded us how overwhelming nature is. The transcendent backdrop of the ocean, autumn colors, and panoramic views from the mountaintops in the park were the perfect settings to rejoice and prepare us for our time with Cybele. Nature—filled with splendor and magnificence—is unparalleled except, perhaps, by the joy of a new grandchild.

Native Americans and indigenous people all around the world went to water or the mountains for spiritual healing and rebirth. Acadia has both. We decided hiking would best help us engage the glory of nature. But first we rested; neither of us had the energy or inclination to hop to it right away. After sleeping late and enjoying a leisurely breakfast, we drove around the park, not stopping much because of the Presidents' Day crowds. Still, the pleasant ride met our need to get the lay of the land. We accomplished our goal to find a place to hike. When Audrey asked a friendly bartender to recommend what shouldn't be missed while in Acadia, without hesitation he said the Beehive Trail on Gorham Mountain, which winds down to Sand Beach—mountain to water.

We set off midmorning the following day. This was our first hike in years, and we were excited. Our scheduled trip to Yosemite during the summer of 2011 had been canceled—one of the casualties of renal failure. For years it was our practice to go to national parks in the Rocky Mountains: Grand Teton, Glacier, and Banff. We learned to enjoy hiking and developed a basic competence at it.

Starting our hike on Gorham Mountain that morning, we felt like tenderfoots. My legs were wobbly and unsteady. The first part of the trail was lined with rocks and small boulders that required stepping or jumping from one to another. For as long as I could remember, I always loved doing this. In my youth, I was a mountain goat. Ordinarily I was extremely confident about my balance and leg strength, feeling I could overcome any difficulty that might present itself. But as I confronted this trail, I found myself very tentative, wondering if I were ready or able for this kind of effort. Fortunately, the trail leveled off and the rocky, stone-strewn path was replaced by the most gorgeous shelves of granite and sandstone that created a natural sidewalk. It reminded me of the terrain in the movie *The Last of the Mohicans*. Making myself available to the experience, my confidence emerged, then grew. When I relaxed, I felt stronger. I saw the beauty of the surroundings. The colors were vibrant and amazing. It was a perfect autumn day, cool but with a warming sun. I was rejuvenated. Audrey reminded me that I couldn't have done this a year ago. Immediately, my awareness was flooded with the significance of what I was doing. The hike validated how far I'd come. My eyes watered as I paused to take in the meaning of what was happening.

When we reached the summit of Gorham Mountain, I was astounded with the beauty and the power of the view. Gratitude, wonder, and humility filled me. Audrey concurred. We were having a moment, a spiritual experience. I had a strong sense of connection with everything around me. The Atlantic Ocean was on our left and the splendid fall colors of Acadia National Park were on our right. In all my life and all our travels, I don't think I'd ever seen a more stunning and breathtaking panorama. This moment was one of intense pleasure and triumph. Climbing Gorham Mountain, albeit only five hundred thirty feet high, was emblematic of my experience for the last twenty-two months. As we drank in the surroundings and felt the pristine power of the experience, I felt healed and restored in full. My life, now richer and fuller, was given back to me. It was only fitting that Audrey and I shared this "holy" moment.

We took almost two more hours to finish the hike, savoring this moment of happiness and peace. We laughed and joked. We paid homage to what had happened over time and in the moment as well. As we continued our descent, we chose a more challenging path, and we traversed it with confidence. Our successful navigation of the rocks, which required scrambling on hands and knees, was deliberate. We felt strong. By the time we reached the oceanfront path and eventually Sand Beach, we were giddy. We'd come full circle. We were back to where we'd started, literally and figuratively.

Then we drove to Cadillac Mountain, thirty minutes away. We declared to our friends and family that we had summited two mountains in one day. We laughed at ourselves and the license we were taking—no sense in being overly serious. Clearly the celebration of my anniversary was off and running.

Two days later, reveling in the memories of our wonderful adventure, we left Maine for Washington, DC. Cybele awaited us.

We hadn't seen our granddaughter in four weeks. She'd changed significantly. The very sight of her filled me with joy and humility like the mountain and ocean, but at an even more profound level. Being in her presence and having a sense of what she represented in my life was overpowering. Cybele entered the world at a moment when my world had been dramatically altered. Her arrival demonstrated incredible timing by the universe—and Sarah. Cybele was simply a miracle, an affirmation of life. Life persists, regenerates, and progresses; it's unstoppable, no matter what human tragedies intervene. The earlier suffering and fear we'd experienced brought us to an even more powerful sense of life and living. In this instance, truth and beauty were packaged in this warm and cuddly eight-pound little girl.

We spent the next few days enjoying Cybele, Sarah, and Chris. Sarah, Cybele, Audrey, and I walked every day somewhere in or near Washington, DC. On the actual anniversary date of my surgery, we found ourselves in Great Falls Park in Virginia. It was only about a thirty-minute drive past Georgetown from the Capitol Hill area, from where Sarah lived at the time. The park, which is my favorite place in the DC area, is at the upper Potomac Falls. I always marvel at how the intense urban pressure of DC can be relieved by traveling just a few miles. This gorgeous spot is where the Potomac River drops eighty-five feet through water-formed crevices, creating rushing falls and breathtaking views. If you walk out onto Olmsted Island, you see the Potomac River, which is slow and meandering in DC but storms through these cliff-lined falls. I'd been there a half a dozen times before, but never with Cybele or on such a momentous occasion. What an impeccable way to celebrate my triumph.

At dinner we toasted my anniversary, and after dinner we called Bret. I texted him the night before, reminding him that one year ago we were applying antibacterial soap all over our bodies in preparation for surgery the next day. During the anniversary call I thanked him, told him I loved him, and reminded him again how he'd changed my life and my families' lives too. He simply said, as he always did, "Thanks" back to me. When I passed the phone to Sarah and Audrey, they also thanked him. When Audrey finally hung up the phone, she said Bret told her, "Enough already. I only gave him a kidney." *What do you say after that?*

We left DC feeling emotionally gratified, but glad to return to the peace and quiet of our regular routine. We'd sufficiently celebrated the landmark moment of our journey. Even knowing more challenges would surely come, we basked in the triumph of crossing the one-year finish line. The sense of completion and triumph and humility remains with me today. These feelings are easily accessible whenever I need to recall my experience and ground myself in the wonder of it all.

Bret's words keep coming back to me as I arrive at the end of my story: "Enough already. I only gave him a kidney." This unpretentious, humble utterance sums him up exquisitely. For Bret, minimalist that he is, donation was only about giving away an extra kidney . . . after all, he had two. For me, his gift encompassed life and love and salvation. Both perspectives are true. And neither exists without the other.

EPILOGUE

LEARNINGS, MUSINGS, AND REFLECTIONS

Perhaps everything terrifying is, in its deepest being, something helpless that wants help from us.

—Rainer Maria Rilke

My life has been immeasurably enriched by my kidney transplant. The experience was so vast, so much more challenging—even fulfilling—than I could have anticipated when my transplant journey started. Making sense of it, interpreting its meaning, is an ongoing process, but here are some reflections I'd like to share.

My transplant experience reinforced how essential *giving* and *generosity* are to living fully. After what I lived through, these concepts are cemented in my mind and soul, and they're central to my story. The capacities to give and to be generous are indispensable to the human spirit. Exercising these characteristics, in my opinion, can even balance the darker parts of the human character, e.g., hate and aggression. This belief was supported by the altruism displayed by Bret and the others who offered to donate. My second chance at life is possible thanks to Bret's exceptional capacity to help me. Hopefully, telling my story will reinforce your belief in the transformative power of giving and generosity.

When individuals (and their circle of friends and family) are confronted with a life-threatening disease such as end-stage renal disease, keeping an open heart and mind rises above all else as critical to coping with and surviving the crisis. Tunneling through anxiety and fear to see beyond it sounds counterintuitive, I know. As someone who lives to tell the tale, I can report a powerful instinct to constrict when everything around you comes undone and fear dominates. Shrinking inward to avoid catastrophe was certainly a strong, almost ever-present temptation. It feels paradoxical to meet overwhelming terror and uncertainty by welcoming it into your life as an opportunity. I didn't want a life-threatening disease that resulted in renal failure; but when it appeared, I chose to believe something could be learned from it. Changing my perspective to view my circumstances not only as a problem to be solved, but as a challenge to engage brought many unexpected gifts. What I initially perceived as an enemy became another life discovery: when our body fails, we must struggle to live. Instead of "circling the wagons" in defense, I learned to engage the threat by staying open to immediate experience, wherever it landed on the spectrum from unremarkable to extraordinary. These attitudes strengthened during my twenty-two-month adventure as I realized that remaining open and flexible generated more paths to survival.

In those first days, weeks, and months of my transplant journey the love I was shown built its own momentum. The more conscious I was of the power of love, the more my heart was pried open. My spirit was nurtured, first by my family and then by my circle of friends. As loving support expanded around me, I understood more firmly that my journey involved more than just surviving PKD and a transplant. I was experiencing an awe-inspiring sense of unconditional love.

The most transparent reason to open my heart was to fight the fear that dominated the situation. If I shut down or closed myself off,

I would have missed that profound gift—unconditional love—offered to me. Fortunately, I learned to take into my heart what was offered. Admittedly, that lesson was absorbed on the fly. Little by little I learned to trust the process. Keeping my heart open wasn't planned, or even consistent, at first. I wasn't noble or wise or self-actualized. I was terrified. I continually felt a strong tidal pull to shut down and protect myself. But I learned. I became more persistent about implementing my newly discovered attitudes. As a result, the paralysis created by fear was kept at bay. Over time the amount of love and support surrounding me was so prodigious that my consciousness expanded. As my trust in this open stance grew, I felt more alive than ever before. The lesson I gleaned: even when staring down the potential for the worst-possible physical outcome, it's far better to see the big-picture good than to focus only on the physical experience of illness and the emotional experience of fear.

Years before my medical crisis, I had embraced the idea of an open mind, or *beginner's mind*, as Laurence Gonzales terms it in the preface of one of my favorite books, *Deep Survival: Who Lives, Who Dies, and Why*. Gonzales is a renowned researcher, lecturer, and author who analyses the data of survivors and writes about who lives and who dies in dramatic, life-threatening situations and accidents: plane crashes, sinking boats, mountain-climbing accidents, and raft trips gone bad. In *Deep Survival*, he draws several conclusions about how and why some individuals survive and some don't. Having always been intrigued by survival stories, this book fascinated me. And during my transplant journey, I came to believe his insights into human behavior apply to situations other than accidents and emergencies. While the urgency quotient may differ, all life-threatening situations—from unforeseen catastrophic accidents to extended illnesses— appear to have similar emotional impact on the individual going through the experience and, consequently, similar approaches can be used to meet the situation.

While immersed in unconditional love and support from friends and family, I began to see the potential to gain even more by examining my attitudes and beliefs. If opening my heart paid such marvelous dividends, what would happen if I also opened my mind to the challenges and struggles? A beginner's mind free—i.e., a mind free of assumptions—allowed me to see the situation as new, which this life-threatening crisis was. Having a beginner's mind limited the intrusion of old, repetitive thoughts and emotions in a survival situation, when lessons learned in previous experiences can interfere with our ability to successfully navigate the threat. An open mind is a straightforward idea, but it's difficult to develop and establish. Doing so turned my focus to asking, *What are the best ways to meet the immense challenge confronting me?* Cultivating this attitude helped me shift from panic to summoning my strength and ability to face the challenge.

In a section of *Deep Survival* called "The Rules of Adventure," Gonzales identifies a dozen concepts that crystallize "how survivors think and behave in the clutch of mortal danger." He offers a how-to guide for survival when faced with catastrophe or a life-threatening situation. His blueprint begins with perceiving the reality of your current situation; moves through staying calm, getting organized, and completing small tasks; lands firmly on believing you'll succeed; and concludes with an admonition to never give up. Having kidney transplant surgery as the result of a lifelong genetic disease certainly warrants using any and all available principles of survival . . . and I did. Applying Gonzales's "rules" to my medical crisis proved extremely useful. I encourage all to read and/or familiarize yourself with these concepts and apply them when you are forced to confront a life-threatening crisis.

For example, *staying calm* helped me confront the ongoing fear of renal failure, transplant surgery, or any serious or life-threatening disease or illness; working to reset to a state of calm as quickly as possible is the best strategy. My bouts with anxiety began in those first days and weeks after end-stage renal disease was confirmed. Later, anxiety hit me like a sledgehammer when possible donors were rejected.

Staying calm during my transplant journey directly correlated to surrendering control. The more I came to terms with surrender, the better able I was to stay calm. Realizing that I couldn't control anything but my own behavior and attitude, and then learning to let go of my need to control, created resilience and strength. Surrendering to surgery and what might happen afterward was the pinnacle of relinquishing control. When surrender became the focus of my experience, relief followed. The practice of truly surrendering must be done without the interfering influences of expectation or pressure toward the desired outcome. In other words, accepting the process takes over and becomes the focus. Whenever I was able to let go, peacefulness returned, and a sense of inner fortitude grew. In fact, the ability to surrender increased exponentially as I used it more frequently. I came to understand that control is an illusion. True surrender requires releasing yourself from the arrogance of control; it's also a bold act of humility. As Gonzales articulates, "To experience humility is the true survivor's correct response to catastrophe."

Integrating Gonzales's rules into my attitude and approach to the problems confronting me led to using more of them: taking correct, decisive action; celebrating my successes; counting my blessings; believing I would succeed; doing whatever is necessary to succeed; never giving up; and living the now. These precepts profoundly affected my action and attitudes.

As those first hours passed in the ICU after the transplant, Audrey helped me make a pivotal realization: being passive in any way during my recovery was unacceptable. Together, as we had at the beginning of our search for a donor, we resolutely committed to do whatever was necessary. By the time Dr. Chon told me I had to take care of the "pristine kidney" I had been given, I was fully dedicated to not just surviving, but thriving. One of the wonderful aspects of this steadfast passion was that it provided a singular focus. Doing whatever was necessary and carrying on were, for the next three months, the only things I had to do—get better, heal, and recover. Not giving up is the most fundamental task of living, and essential during a crisis. I firmly believed this credo most of my life, but certainly now as an adult in my situation. It is an exquisite and elegant notion that should be adopted early in a transplant adventure. The commitment to this attitude empowers you during the struggle and keeps the door to survival open.

Another key discovery of my transplant journey emerged during my recovery as I learned how the renewal of the body can have significant spiritual repercussions. Inspired by Gonzales's reminder to count your blessings, the more gratitude I embraced, the better I felt, the faster I healed, and the more thankful I became. In an interesting convergence, this transition coincided with my reading of *The Spirituality of Imperfection* by Ernest Kurtz and Katherine Ketcham. During my recovery, their book provided a structure and inspiration for framing my experience beyond the physical. It helped me examine what it meant to receive an organ from another person and then have it keep me alive. I can't emphasize enough the strange, even eerie, quality of having Bret's kidney and how it impacts the way I live. I struggled daily with the question: *Why did this happen to me?* Working to answer that altered my perception of not only what I was experiencing, but the very essence of my life. The nature of my expansive experience required a new mental framework to begin the arduous task of making sense of it all.

Struggling with and then surviving a crisis offers a simple clarity. Although I felt surrounded by innumerable complexities, the two things at the core of my story were *survival* and *getting better*. To narrow down the complicated act of living to the fundamental act of staying alive is a gift in and of itself. My focus sharpened; distractions shrunk. I was often living minute to minute, even second to second, if pain was present, and no more than day to day in the big picture of recovery. Life in recovery moved rapidly and was relentless. A bad moment was replaced by a wonderful one. Never was I so fundamentally alive as during this time.

As my recovery unfolded, I eventually accepted that I was going to live, which meant moving forward with a new kidney. One of the nephrologists who worked with my sister told her that having someone else's organ inside of you *isn't natural*. These words had a deep impact on me, hitting home in those early days and throughout my recovery. The anachronism of transforming an inherently "unnatural" occurrence into my body's new status quo was a daunting task.

Adjusting to this new, earth-shattering reality kindled my intense gratitude. I'm acutely aware of how fortunate I was to find a living donor and receive a perfect kidney from an incredibly healthy, young individual. When I consider the possibility that my good fortune was the result of only randomness, I get weak in the knees. *Could randomness alone explain good fortune?* If true, it would be even more overwhelming. But it's possible. Scientists or certain philosophers might support this point of view. But for me, it doesn't singularly satisfy or enlighten my experience. Also, because I'm not religious, I can't entirely explain my transplant experience as the result of spiritual forces intervening and giving me this incredible gift. Neither chance nor a guiding spirit offers an adequate explanation for what transpired. I've come to believe a synergistic combination of chance, the power of the human spirit (as exercised through being proactive, keeping an open heart and mind, and maintaining a positive attitude), and unexplained spiritual or energetic forces help explain my experience. Why not a combination of forces in our control and those out of our scope? And in the end, perhaps no explanation is truly necessary—or possible. Acceptance and wonder may be enough.

Experiencing the level of good fortune and grace I did made it easier to see the beauty in other situations. Essential to the transcendent beauty of my transplant journey was the outpouring of unconditional love and support from the people who reached out to me via CaringBridge. Never in my life had I experienced love and support at this volume and intensity—and it went right to my heart. In a CaringBridge entry I described my experience as a series of "truth and beauty moments," and those words still feel accurate. In those early days and weeks of recovery, I felt sustained and carried by these moments. Regardless of the physical outcome of the surgery, including rejection of the kidney, I knew I'd already received life's most beautiful gift. My heart expanded as a result—surely that's an unexpected outcome of renal failure and kidney transplant surgery. I learned through experience that fear and ecstasy can exist simultaneously.

The most rewarding experiences in my life—whether they were part of teaching or relationships or parenting or merely part of exploring who I was and how I wanted to live—all included an element of *egolessness*. In those memorable moments, I stayed out of my own way and made myself available to the energy of the experience itself, to both share and receive. Diminishing my ego as best I could, whenever I could, enhanced my awareness and allowed me to absorb the many gifts bestowed upon me during the transplant process. Humility is a gift and a practice. I can say without hesitation that I am a better human for having gone through this challenging, scary, and incredible experience than I was before it. My life is richer and fuller now. I vividly learned facing a crisis or life-threatening situation, of any kind, is merely a part of living. Focusing on living during my challenge was what became most important to me. I invite you to do the same.

I can't emphasize enough how fortunate I was throughout my journey. So many things, so often, broke my way. Windfalls seemed to compound each other. My transplant story is a privileged one— physically, emotionally, and spiritually. Many others have not fared as well and, consequently, would have a different story to tell or a different message for the reader. All I can do is share my experience as honestly as possible. And although I don't wish a medical crisis on anyone, I am better for having experienced one.

Here are some things I discovered along the way. I offer them to you from a survivor's perspective. I hope they may help you as you navigate your life journeys:

1. Living demands courage.

2. Vulnerability is not weakness but rather leads to courage.

3. Surviving and success, however they're measured, result from facing adversity rather than trying to avoid it.

4. Your attitude toward adversity is of utmost importance.

5. Support and love are essential. Surrounding yourself with people who love you makes all the difference.

6. Adapting to change is a constant.

7. Patience serves you and those around you well.

8. Being proactive and persevering contributes to a positive outcome.

9. The sheer power of giving is astounding.

10. Unconditional love heals.

11. Seeing your condition as a challenge rather than a problem helps you cope and even flourish.

12. Altruism authentically opens the human heart and allows healing to happen.

13. Having an open heart and mind boosts your creativity and makes you a better problem solver.

14. Accepting ambiguity is a key step in confronting a medical crisis.

15. Control, particularly of the outcome, is an illusion, so surrender and let go whenever possible.

16. Keep perspective. Strive to leave your ego behind. Don't just focus on yourself; engage others and stay aware of what else is happening around you and in the world. Life goes on no matter what happens to you.

17. Embrace humility.

My words (any words, really) fall short in describing the force and power of my experience. Even reaching this point of identifying and articulating them with a measure of clarity feels hard won. I paid a steep emotional price to acquire this understanding of my transplant experience. As one gesture of paying it forward, I offer this attempt to distill what I've discovered as a gift to you. May this book help you learn, survive, and flourish despite the challenges you face. And may you discover the same kind of gratitude I've had the privilege to embrace.

ACKNOWLEDGMENTS

So many people require my gratitude and acknowledgement.

Audrey sits at the summit of the mountain of light and love. I wouldn't be here without her. She forever has my unfaltering gratitude.

I am powerfully grateful that my family was thoroughly devoted during my entire story. Sarah, Emily, and Luke exemplified support and unconditional love. Thank you for being there for me.

A special note of appreciation and love to my sons-in-law: Chris Fickes and Terry Parmelee. Your steadfast compassion and support of Sarah and Emily, respectively, were truly acts of love and beauty. Your behavior during our family crisis speaks to your dignity and integrity. And the kindness you displayed toward me and Audrey puts you in the Sons-In-Law Hall of Fame.

My wonderful extended family members—Roseann, Jerry, Bill and Irene, Ken and Sharon—were indispensable with their encouragement, support, and humor. Thank you for filling my heart and keeping me going.

My amazing and wonderful would-be donors who tried but couldn't cross the finish line: John, Roseann, and Ken. Heroes you were, heroes you are. Your goodness still endures in me.

To those who offered to donate a kidney to me—Al Downs, Randy Zatrock, Majid Ghadiri, my nephew Mike Baldauf, Susan Eriksen, and even a stranger I met at lunch and whose name I've long forgotten. Please know your goodness and amazing offers helped sustain me and your caring act still resides in my heart.

I want to acknowledge and honor the donors in my extended family. My second cousin Cathy Jorgensen gave a kidney to my aunt Marge Bencivenga. Another second cousin, Paul May, gave a kidney to my cousin Sharon Gitzen. And in 2017 Paul's sister, Patty May, gave her kidney to my first cousin Jack Baldauf (Sharon's brother). Astounding goodness must run in our family. Cathy, your gift led the way and lit the path for our extended family to follow. Along with your kidneys, the three of you gave and renewed life. From the heart, thank you for your generosity, and for giving us all the gift of hope.

I was surprised at how my friends kept showing up and staying. Alan and Patty Rubin, who were there from the beginning and stayed throughout, embodied goodness and grace. Your kind caring actions are to be marveled at. You are the poster children for good friends. Bernie and Susan Silver came to the hospital the day of the transplant, and even stayed in Chicago longer before leaving for Florida to see that I was all right. Their visit the day before their departure was an act of kindness I'll never forget. Smokey and Elaine Daniels, I counted on and looked forward to your continuous care and concern. Jim and Ellen Bush were constant presences in my heart during my struggle. Other old friends—Jack and Claudia Steinberg and Margaret Hershey—helped me through my crisis, even from afar. Margaret, your late-night post the night of the transplant surgery still resonates in my heart.

My friends continued to be an integral part of my long recovery. I anticipated, to a certain extent, their compassion before the transplant surgery, but not necessarily after it. The quantity and intensity of how people attended to me while I was in need over time astounded me. I'm deeply thankful. It was essential to my recovery. Kevin Fitzpatrick and Wendy Kopald are at the top of the list. Your visits after my surgery are still remembered.

Of special note are the Knuckleheads—Cary Schawel, Paul Johnson, Joe Kotowski, and Jan Thompson-Wilda—who changed the meaning of what work friends are and exceeded those boundaries. Thank you for daily sustaining me, without fail, at work and beyond. Wow.

Practically speaking and in its most basic form, my success came down to the skill of my surgeon, Dr. Yolanda Becker. How lucky I was that you did the transplant surgery. I'm glad you chose medicine and not the violin as your career path. Thank you, thank you, thank you.

Thank you to the marvelous medical staff—with a special nod to the nurses Mary Beth, Roseann, and Jo—at UChicago's Transplant Clinic. You're amazing. You guided me through the perilous waters of recovery with skill, grace, and empathy. Who knew three angels would see me through my adventure? Kudos to you and your marvelous professionalism.

Dr. James Chon and all the others at the clinic, I trusted your skill and knowledge. It made me feel safe. Please know I am still taking wonderful care of the "pristine" kidney Bret gave me.

Dr. Kevin Nash, your care before I went into renal failure was fantastic—and when I went into end-stage renal disease, you were amazing. You kept your promise to help keep me off dialysis. Your help during my Christmas ER visit was so important, and your care following my release from the transplant clinic was exquisite.

Joi Smith and Peg Lee, you eased my mind at work and gave me your blessing to recover at my own pace. You were both classy and caring—and exemplary administrators who put in action how a leader should be.

Years after my transplant, several people I trusted read my manuscript and gave me wonderful feedback on it: Audrey, Emily, Roseann, Irene, Elaine and Smokey Daniels, Paul Johnson, Jack Steinberg, Jim Bush, Dick Gardner, Alan and Patricia Rubin, Bernie Silver, and Susan Eriksen. Thank you for your insight and care; it significantly helped me move the project down the road.

Smokey Daniels, thank you for being the impetus to get what I wrote to a publishing company. Your wisdom and knowledge were essential to finally making the book happen and bringing my words to a conclusion. Your review and feedback, particularly while you were dealing with a family medical crisis, makes what you did even more amazing. You rock, man.

To the wonderful people at Beaver's Pond Press. You folks are great. Alicia, you have a gift for guiding fledging, nonprofessional would-be writers like me. Grace and enthusiasm are yours.

Of special note is Wendy Weckwerth, my editor. You're marvelous. How patient, kind, and powerful a teacher you are. You made my writing and the telling of my story so much better. I can't thank you enough for your work . . . and I love you for it.

To all those who took the time to express their concern and care on the CaringBridge site, I thank you. You became an integral and intimate part of my life. The entries highlighted my experience and elicited glorious feelings of love, joy, and humility. Being the recipient of such love and care and humor left me stunned and humbled. *Humbling gratitude* is what I felt for all who participated. Your generous and compassionate words had a profound effect on my healing and recovery. You were my heroes every day. I remain grateful for your participation in my adventure.

RESOURCES AND DONATION

Please consider giving to one of the following organizations working toward a cure for PKD. Your donations can support research and patient and family education that will impact the experiences of those in need of a kidney transplant. You have the power to make a difference in so many lives. I urge you to help.

All profits from the sale of this book will be distributed to nonprofit organizations working to find a cure for PKD. Additionally, part of the proceeds will be donated to a college fund established for Bret's children, Hadley and Brinley.

PKD Foundation (Polycystic Kidney Disease Foundation)
1001 East 101st Terrace, Suite 220
Kansas City, MO 64131
1-800-PKD-CURE (1-800-753-2873)
pkdcure.org

National Kidney Foundation (NKF)
30 East 33rd Street
New York, NY 10016
1-800-622-9010
kidney.org

American Association of Kidney Patients (AAKP)
14440 Bruce B. Downs Boulevard
Tampa, FL 33613
1-800-749-2257
aakp.org

For information on becoming a living donor, see the Organ Donation and Transplantation section of the NKF website, kidney.org. Of particular interest is NKF's Living Donor Council, which was formed to support those considering living donation.

The Living Bank
4545 Oak Place Drive, Suite 340
Houston, TX 77027
1-800-528-2971
livingbank.org

Organ Procurement and Transplantation Network (OPTN)
P.O. Box 2484
Richmond, VA 23218
optn.transplant.hrsa.gov

National Living Donor Assitance (NLDAC)
1401 South Clark Street, Suite 120
Arlington, VA 22202
888-670-5002
livingdonorassistance.org

ABOUT THE AUTHOR

Greg Baldauf was born in Chicago and lived there for most of his life, eventually raising a family with his wife, Audrey, in Evanston, a northern suburb. After completing an undergraduate degree at Northwestern University, he briefly taught high school English in downstate Marion, Illinois. Returning to Chicago, Greg did graduate work in counseling at Loyola University. While completing a PhD in counseling psychology, he was hired and eventually became a professor of psychology and student development at Oakton Community College in Des Plaines, Illinois. In his thirty-one years at Oakton, Greg studied and taught wellness, men's psychology, topics in human services, and substance-abuse counseling. He also explored aspects of multicultural psychology and spirituality through the study of Incan shamanism and working with Andean medicine people in Peru.

Greg is the father of three wonderful children who play an essential role in his story. He's now humbled and fortunate to have three amazing grandchildren: Cybele, Stella, and Graham. Now retired, Greg and Audrey live in Venice, Florida.